your

# SAVE^ FACE

## The Truth About Facial Aging, Its Prevention and "Cure"

## Brooke Rutledge Seckel, M.D.

Assistant Professor of Surgery
Harvard Medical School

First Edition

Peach Publications • Concord, Massachusetts

your

# SAVE ^ FACE

## The Truth About Facial Aging, Its Prevention and "Cure"

**By Brooke Rutledge Seckel, M.D.**

## IMPORTANT-PLEASE READ

**Limit of Liability/Disclaimer of Warranty:** This book is written as a source of information and for educational purposes only and is not intended to be complete or exhaustive. The information in this book is not intended as a replacement for the advice of a qualified medical professional. A qualified medical professional should always be consulted before beginning any diet, medication, nutritional protocol, vitamin, mineral, herbal product, hormone supplement, and similar preparations, exercise, lifestyle modification, surgical procedure, remedy, skin care, or any anti-aging or other procedure or protocol mentioned in this book. Any use of the information in this book is at the reader's discretion. Every effort has been made to ensure the accuracy of the information contained in this book as of the date of publication. Neither the author nor publisher advocate the use of any particular health-care protocol, but believe that the information in this book should be available to the public. The author and publisher specifically disclaim any and all liability arising directly or indirectly from the use or application of any information contained in this book.

Published by Peach Publications, Inc., Concord, Massachusetts
No part of this publication may be reproduced, stored in a retrieval system, or transmitted in any form or by any means, electronic, mechanical, photocopying, recording, scanning, or otherwise without the written permission of the author except for brief quotations used in a review or critical article.

For information about this and other products call 1-866-352-3222 or visit http://saveyourface.com

**Publisher's Cataloging-in-Publication**
Seckel, Brooke R.
Save your face: the truth about facial aging, its
prevention and "cure" / Brooke Rutledge Seckel. -- 1st Ed.
P. cm.
Includes bibliographical references and index.
The word "your" appears as an inserted word between
"Save" and "face" on t.p.
LCCN 2005900873
ISBN 0-9765518-0-2
ISBN 0-9765518-1-0
1. Face--Care and hygiene.
2. Face--Aging.
3. Beauty, Personal.    I. Title.
RL87.S38 2005                646.7'26
QBI05-200036

# The Peach: Chinese Symbol of Longevity

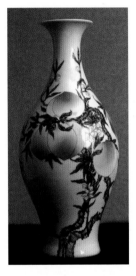

The inspiration for the cover of this book came from the beautiful peach motifs which are so often found on old Chinese pottery and porcelain. In Chinese folklore the peach is the symbol of longevity and immortality. The peach is considered a sacred fruit which grows on a special tree near the palace of Xiwangmu. Xiwangmu is Queen of the immortals and the peach tree near her palace blooms every 3000 years. Anyone who eats the fruit of this tree gains immortality.

I love the beauty of the peach but also present it to my readers in the hope that by reading this book they will partake of the peach and gain healthy longevity

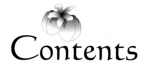

# Contents

# Chapter 4 **85**

## HOW TO SAVE YOUR FACE – FEED YOUR MIND, BODY, AND SPIRIT **85**

# Chapter 5     **125**

## HOW TO REVERSE FACIAL AGING –
## DOCTOR SECKEL'S 6-STEP PROGRAM   **125**

# Chapter 6     **133**

## MAGICAL POTIONS –
## THE FOUNTAIN OF YOUTH   **133**

# Chapter 7      159

## NO DOWN TIME FACIAL ANTI-AGING PROCEDURES      159

# Chapter 8      189

## HIGH-TECH FACIAL REJUVENATION: LASERS, INTENSE PULSED LIGHT (IPL), INFRARED LIGHT (TITAN®), RADIOFREQUENCY (THERMAGE®), AND LED (GENTLEWAVES®) – NON-ABLATIVE THERAPIES      189

To

Tommy and Laura
My Joy and Inspiration

Robert and Kathy
My Friends

And

Martha
My Guardian Angel

# Acknowledgements

Kathleen Burke not only provided superb illustrations for this book but also served as copy editor, proof-reader, promoter, public relations officer, and design consultant. More importantly her close friendship and support throughout this entire project have played an essential role in its completion.

I express my deepest thanks to Diane Bair, editor, Maria Fernanda Gamba, cover design and typesetting, Gilberto Gamba and Rick Chevalier, photo editing, and Melinda Steadman, manuscript preparation.

I am blessed to be surrounded by a large group of professionals who provide daily support to me in my plastic surgery practice both in my office and the operating room. Without the kind and caring support of these individuals the task of writing this book would have been much more difficult. Janice Ianone, Dawn O'Toole, Amy Defeo, Barbara Spracklin, Sheryl Scannel, Monique LeBlanc, Carolyn Newall, Mary Reed, Melinda Steadman, Amy Guertin, Ann Tobin, Ann Twomey, and Donna Hall all are valued friends and associates whose kind support enables me to fulfill my multifaceted mission.

Finally, I am truly blessed and privileged to be a plastic surgeon for my many patients whose emotional feedback and trust have inspired me to continue looking for a better way to practice my profession. I am so grateful to them all.

**Brooke R. Seckel, M.D.**

# About The Author

Dr. Brooke R. Seckel is a nationally and internationally recognized authority in Plastic Surgery and the treatment of facial aging. He performs all types of cosmetic, facial and breast plastic surgery, but his special interest lies in the field of non-invasive and non-surgical therapies to correct and prevent facial aging.

Dr. Seckel is founder and Director of the Lahey Center for Cosmetic and Laser Surgery in Lexington, Massachusetts. He was the first chairman of the Department of Plastic Surgery at The Lahey Clinic in Burlington, Massachusetts, a large multi-specialty group practice hospital in the Boston area.

He is certified by the American Board of Plastic Surgery, is a member of the American Society of Plastic Surgery, The American Society for Aesthetic Plastic Surgery, the Boston Surgical Society, is an Assistant Professor of Surgery at Harvard Medical School, and was recently honored by his peers by being voted one of the "Best Doctors in America".

Dr. Seckel has published over one hundred scientific articles in the field of plastic surgery and authored the first book on cosmetic laser surgery entitled "Aesthetic Laser Surgery". He is also a Board Certified Neurologist and published "Facial Danger Zones", a book devoted to teaching surgeons how to perform facial surgery safely without injuring the facial nerves.

Dr. Seckel founded and served as Program Director of the Lahey Clinic Residency Program in Plastic Surgery. He has taught for many years that with advances in technology Plastic Surgery is becoming less "surgical" and more of a preventative discipline. The exciting advances in the field of anti-aging medicine during the past ten years have prompted Dr. Seckel to write this book in which he presents a comprehensive preventative and therapeutic approach to the timely topic of facial rejuvenation

Dr. Seckel resides in Concord, Massachusetts and is the father of Laura and Tommy Seckel. In his spare time he enjoys sailing on Cape Cod, woodworking, building furniture, wooden boat restoration, restoring his antique home and jogging with his German Shepard, Griffin.

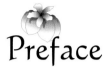

# Preface

I have been a physician for 35 years and a plastic surgeon for the past 23. Personally, there are few joys that match sharing the happiness and enthusiasm of seeing one of my patients look into a mirror following plastic surgery. They see a face they remember, happily, from the past – a young face, a smiling face, a face looking ahead to the possibilities and dreams of the future. For me, plastic surgery is all about empowerment, about helping people realize their potential as human beings. Unfortunately, the effects of the aging process, which have been going on since the day we were born, become dramatically visible first on our face long before our mind, body, and spirit are willing to accept the notion that "that's all there is."

While some say we should "grow old gracefully," my experience as a doctor (not to mention the recent explosion in the field of anti-aging medicine), reveals that baby boomers do not accept this irrelevant, outdated concept.

Aging transforms the face to create a tired, fatigued, drawn look that belies the essence of the person inside. Contemporary American society seems reluctant to acknowledge the fact that, behind an aging face, is a vibrant person with the same visions, fantasies, goals, desires and needs of a younger person just starting adult life.

Sadly, for our society and for mankind, these changes are most apparent and most striking at a time in our lives when we have reached our greatest potential as human beings. In our middle years, we're enriched with the knowledge and wisdom gained through our experiences, so we approach the important events of life with a much more effective problem solving strategy than we could when we were younger and less experienced. Our skills and our vitality, enhanced with our own strength and maturity, can improve the human experience for all.

What does looking younger have to do with such far-reaching and profound concepts?

There are at least two very important benefits to maintaining a youthful appearance. First, your appearance has a profound effect on your self-esteem, which is a major factor effecting your mood, enthusiasm, and energy, factors which empower you to live a productive and fulfilling life. Secondly, for better or for worse, our youth-oriented, fast-paced, competitive, Madison Avenue dominated culture promotes and values a youthful appearance over old.

This prejudice often impacts our careers and social lives in an inhibitory and harmful way. Loss of career opportunity and social relevance are particularly devastating to our sense of well – being, especially in a society in which traditional, long-term, mutually supportive relationships such as marriage and long-term employment at one company have ceased to be the norm.

I will not argue with those who tell me that my opinions and musings are vanity-based, insecure, and superficial. They are entitled to their view and may have it in peace. My opinions are my own based on my

30 years of experience as a doctor and are affirmed daily by the patients who make up my large and meaningful plastic surgical practice. My patients are wonderful, sane people who understand the issues of aging and have the courage to resist feeling and looking older. They refuse to passively accept what fate has offered to previous generations. History will never describe our generation, the so-called "baby boomer" generation, as passive!

My major concern regarding the current interest in the field of facial aging: Technology is outpacing the ability of doctors to safely incorporate many of the new anti-aging therapies into medical practice. Traditionally, a new medical therapy, like the polio vaccine, was tested and tried in the laboratory until it was proven to be safe and effective for human use. Only then was it made available to those doctors who possessed the knowledge and skills to safely use the new product for the benefit of patients.

The world of health care is a vastly different place today. Many manufacturers of medical equipment have made a conscious decision to focus their business on anti-aging because they perceive the substantial potential for profit in this field. The same corporations have also learned the immense power of marketing. Today, new anti-aging technologies are seductively marketed directly to you the consumer, not the doctor – often, in my opinion, before their effectiveness and safety have been proven. You, the potential patient, get excited by the often-unrealistic marketing claims and demand these treatments from your doctor. The doctor is placed in a difficult position. He or she must pay the corporation for a $50,000 or $100,000 laser to avoid being perceived as being not up to date in the field and, worse, may lose patients to a doctor who already has the new machine. This pattern of behavior reflects corporate arrogance, greed, and lack of concern for the safety and welfare of patients.

Of course, when the therapies do not work, the truth will be known and the product will fail, but only after millions of dollars have changed hands from patient to doctor to corporation. If you doubt me, look on the Internet for advertisements for used medical lasers, $150,000-$200,000 machines available for $5,000-$10,000 "like new." Of course they are new. The machines did not deliver what was promised and were never used. Hopefully, no one was physically hurt during the short time the machines were in service.

Another alarming trend, particularly in the field of facial rejuvenation, is that many of the new anti-aging therapies are being offered to patients by practitioners without medical degrees, in spas and other non-medical centers. This trend is partially due to the fact that many of the new therapies are non-invasive and appear so easy to perform that people assume that anyone can provide these treatments. Then there's the fact that the contemporary medical community has been slow to incorporate new anti-aging therapies into current medical practice-even though, as this book will document, there is substantial credible scientific evidence to support many of the new therapies. Finally, non-physician entrepreneurs have discovered the immense financial potential of the field of facial anti-aging and are eager to cash in on this bonanza without going to medical school and learning to treat patients in an appropriate and safe way.

Regardless of the circumstance, you, the patient are exposed to unnecessary risks when you receive medical therapies from someone other than a knowledgeable and skilled doctor. What happens if some serious medical complication occurs in a spa and there is no doctor present? That's a frightening thought! I predict that the newly evolving "medical spa" with physicians on staff will become the primary source for preventive medical care in the future. The model will be a true HMO or health maintenance organization helping patients prevent illness instead of denying access to medical care as, the current managed care industry is doing in a disgracefully short-sighted manner.

In this book, I will present what I understand to be the truth about the causes, prevention and treatment of facial aging. As a plastic surgeon, I know that we can successfully make your face look 20 or 30 years younger with surgery. The goal, however, is to prevent aging of the face or, if that is not possible, to rejuvenate your face without harming you in the process.

Please be patient while reading this book. There is a great deal of technical information on the following pages. Some of this is not easy reading! But you need to know the facts if you are going to make correct choices. You need to understand the cause before you can go for the cure.

What you learn in this book will empower you to make the right choices and not be fooled by some advertisement that insults your intelligence by promising the fountain of youth, taking your money and leaving you unchanged or worse off than when you started. So relax, sit down with a cup of green tea and some soft music and start reading. It will take some time and effort on your part, but in the end you will be a very powerfully educated consumer in the new anti-aging marketplace.

Why am I writing this book? First, I love to write. Second, I love to teach. Ultimately, it is because, I get great joy in experiencing the beauty of restoration, whether I'm restoring a patient's face, my old wooden boat, or my wonderful 160-year-old home.

Nothing makes me happier than seeing something showing signs of age brought back to gleaming brilliance once again, shining and new but with the glowing patina of depth and quality that only time and experience can produce.

**Brooke R. Seckel, M.D**

Concord, Massachusetts

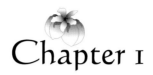

# Chapter 1

# IS THAT MY MOTHER
# I SEE IN THE MIRROR?

All of us reflect our heredity, and nowhere is that reflection more dramatic than in our facial appearance. The most common complaint of my 30 – to 40 – year-old patients when they first seek consultation for facial aging

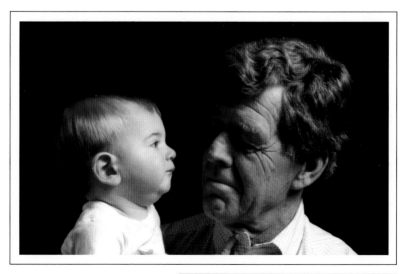

**FIGURE 1-1.**
*The effect of six decades of facial aging on the face we are born with.*

is, "I'm starting to look like my mother" or "father" as the case may be. Of course they have always looked like Mom or Dad, but now they are starting to see wrinkles and other changes that make them resemble their 60- or 70- year-old parent.

Look at the photograph on the previous page (Figure 1-1) and try to understand exactly what it is that makes our face look old. This picture is the first slide in my lecture about plastic surgery for facial aging. It graphically demonstrates the impact of six decades of aging on the face we are all born with.

The baby's skin is smooth, plump, unblemished, moist, radiant, and firm, yet supple and elastic. If you gently pull on the child's cheek and let go, the skin snaps back instantly, a quality we call elasticity. In contrast, the man's skin is rough, dry, with wrinkles and multiple blemishes – brown spots called age spots, and small blood vessels called telangiectasias. There are also red spots with scaly white flaking skin over them called actinic keratoses, spots that may eventually grow into a skin cancer. His skin does not glow like the skin of the infant and the child's healthy radiance has been replaced by a sallow, dull, almost yellowish appearance.

These superficial changes are caused primarily by years of exposure to the sun and other harmful agents in our environment. Doctors refer to these superficial skin changes as Type I facial aging changes. Type I facial aging is most evident on the surface of your skin, the superficial skin layer called the epidermis.

The skin of the man is wrinkled and sagging, with folds of skin hanging on his face. If you grasp his skin with your thumb and index finger and let go, the skin does not snap back like the child's skin. Instead, it takes 5 to 10 seconds to go back to its original shape. This is skin laxity, the hallmark of aged facial skin. These changes are caused by aging damage to the deeper layers of the skin, the dermis, and are called Type II facial aging changes. Type II facial aging changes are the result of our heredity, nutrition, exposure to the sun and other toxins, and lifestyle. The most important skin change that causes Type II facial aging changes is the loss of the elasticity of the skin. The cause of the loss of elasticity: Damage to the collagen and elastin, two important structural proteins present in the dermis or deeper layer of your skin.

All modern facial rejuvenation therapies attempt to correct Type I and Type II facial aging changes. Aging changes in the face are complex and impact different parts of the face in different ways at different times and differently in different people. Let's look at the diagram of the aged face on the next page (Figure 1-2) and analyze the changes in each part of the face.

The left side of this facial diagram shows the end result of six or seven decades of sun damage and aging. I like to analyze the face in thirds: the upper third (forehead and eyes), the middle third (cheeks and nose), and the lower third (mouth, jaw line and neck.) Although the same aging phenomenon is impacting all three areas, the results of facial aging are different in each area and show up at different times in your life. The therapies that correct these aging changes are different for each area. Understanding this concept will help you understand the correctional therapies discussed later in this book.

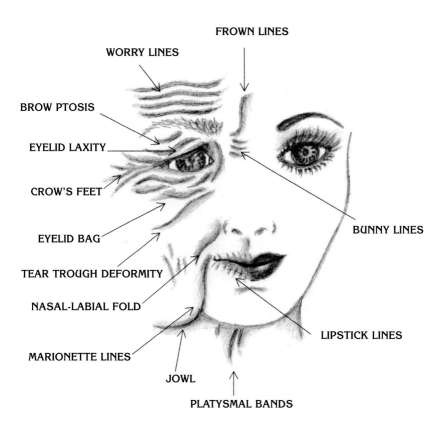

**FIGURE 1-2.**
*Visible facial changes with aging.*

Eyelid changes are the earliest sign of facial aging and are the first to occur in the upper third of the face. These happen in almost all people in their 30's. The earliest changes are wrinkles, **crow's feet, worry lines, frown lines**, and **bunny lines**. These lines are actually caused by the pull of our underlying muscles of facial expression, muscles that function to express our emotions.

Later, the upper eyelid skin begins to sag or droop over the beautiful eyelid fold (called the supratarsal fold) and eventually over the eyelashes themselves. This creates a tired look. The lower eyelid begins to show permanent lines or wrinkles associated with the same muscle pull that is causing the crow's feet. Another lower eyelid change is puffiness or bagginess of the lower eyelid. This is caused by loss of elasticity of the skin and muscle of the eyelid. This allows the fat, which normally lies beneath the eyeball supporting it, to push outward or herniate, a fancy term for a bulge. This change is commonly referred to as **eyelid bags**. There are also textural skin changes in the eyelid that make the skin look old.

There are many non-surgical, topical, laser and other therapies that can remedy the superficial skin changes. However once the deeper changes have occurred in the lower eyelid, plastic surgery is required to correct them. Claiming that a skin cream can significantly correct lax skin and bulging fat in the eyelid is, in my opinion, false advertising! Don't believe it.

Another very striking facial aging change, which involves the upper third and middle third of the face, is called the **tear trough deformity**. It is that sad, oblique line that runs from just under the eyelid, starting at the nose and running out and down the very top of the cheek towards the ear. This is an advanced sign, which typically occurs in the late 50s to 60s, but it often begins in the late 30s or early 40s as a dark circle or shadow beneath the eyelid. This is caused by the fact that your lower eyelid muscle is attached to the bone of your eye socket and it can't fall downward with the eyelid skin as the bulging fat is pushing your eyelid out and down. The result is a deep crease that becomes a shadow under your eyelid. As the cheek starts to fall, the area stays tethered to the bone, which creates an ever-increasing depression and shadow along the line.

Early on, we call this change "dark circles", or "tired look," but later it forms a deep line or trough into which your tears roll out to the side of your face and not straight down you cheek, as they did when you were a child, thus "tear trough deformity."

Now look at the eyebrows of the face in the diagram. The eyebrows has sagged or drooped down over the eye, especially the outer portion on the side of the face nearest the ear. This phenomenon is called **brow ptosis** and is caused not only by loss of elasticity of the skin but also by the sagging of fat, which lies beneath the eyebrow.

There are several major facial aging events occurring in the middle of the face that create an aged appearance. The most profound is the sagging of the cheek, which produces the fold of skin hanging down around the mouth called the **nasal-labial fold**. This aging change is caused by two things: laxity, or the loss of elasticity of the skin and underlying structures of the face (which allows gravity to pull the skin down,) and the fall of the malar fat pad, or cheek fat pad.

As a child, this pad of fat under the cheek skin is attached high up on your cheekbone, just under the eyes. Remember those chubby cheeks that all the grownups like to pinch? Look at your children. They have nice, full cheeks up high on their faces. As we age, the malar fat pad descends into the middle of our cheek. Making things worse are your smile muscles. Look in the mirror and smile. Do you see the smile line? It is caused by a muscle that pulls on the corner of your mouth, pulling your mouth up and out to the side when you smile. The smile line runs from the corner of your nose to the corner of your mouth. Notice how the cheek hangs over this line? The combination of the loss of elasticity (which allows the skin to sag), the downward fall of the malar fat pad, and years of smiling create the deep smile line with the folds of skin hanging over it. We call this aged smile line the **nasal-labial fold line**. The action of the smile muscles also creates wrinkles in the cheek, which become permanent as the skin ages. Also notice that as the malar fat pad has dropped forming the nasal-labial fold, there is a facial depression where it used to be. This depression contributes to the tear trough deformity.

The impact of facial aging has a profound effect on the lower third of the face. Vertical wrinkles called **lipstick lines** develop around the lips fairly early often in the 30s. Smoking horribly accentuates these lines. If you don't smoke, you may never get them, or they will be smaller and less significant. The upper lip also sags due to loss of elasticity and atrophy or wasting away of normal fat inside the lip. As a result, the lip becomes longer. Did you ever hear of the expression "long in the tooth," referring to old people? The pink part of your upper lip, the "Cupid's Bow," becomes thinner and turns downward and inward and the corners of the mouth turn down. The most common complaint I hear is "People think I am angry or mean and I am not." This is especially true when deep frown lines and aging changes around the mouth are present in the same face. The sagging of the cheek, which causes the nasal-labial fold, also causes the skin to fall down over the corner of the mouth and chin to form **marionette lines**. (Remember Mr. Bluster the irritable old man marionette on the puppet show Howdy Doody?) The chin also droops in some people, usually only in the late 50s or 60s, but it is very distressing to those who experience this. The horrible term "witches chin" is used to describe it. (Remember the cartoon character, Hilda the Witch?)

The descent of the facial skin also causes sagging along the jaw line, creating **jowls**. As the neck ages, the neck skin becomes lax and falls into folds below the chin, a deformity referred to as "turkey wattle". Frequently, there are prominent bands on the neck called **platysmal bands** because they are caused by the pull and laxity of the two platysma muscles underneath the chin. These muscles act like cords, pulling the skin folds down along two lines running from under your chin to the middle of your neck.

These changes are what many of you can expect to see at the end of 70 years of facial aging if you do not take steps now to prevent them. But the severity of aging in the face varies, depending on your genetic makeup and how well you take care of yourself. Don't expect face creams to correct these major structural changes, even though this concept is often promoted in the media. Those who fall for this do not understand the complex anatomical changes that occur in the aging face. Fortunately, you're reading this book so you won't be misled. Obviously, you do not want to end up like the person in Figure 2 or you would not have bought this book! I don't want you to end up like that either. Let's move on to Chapter 2 and take a close-up look at what causes these distressing changes to occur in our face. First, let's summarize what we have learned so far in the table on the next page, (Table 1-1).

The age ranges in Table 1 are generalizations. People with Type I and Type II skin, redheads and fair blondes (see Table 3-1, Chapter 3 for skin types) will age earlier at the lower end of the age range. Darker skinned patients will age later. Smokers, drinkers and people with unhealthy lifestyles will age and develop facial wrinkles much earlier.

| Aging Change | When First Seen | Cause | Aging Type | Correctable? |
|---|---|---|---|---|
| Brown Spots "Broken" Blood Vessels Dry, Rough Skin | 28-30 years | Sun and other toxic damage to superficial skin-the epidermis | Type I | Yes |
| Frown Lines | 28-30 years | Pull of facial muscle | Type II | Yes |
| Worry Lines | 28-30 years | Pull of facial muscle | Type II | Yes |
| Crow's Feet | 28-30 years | Pull of facial muscle | Type II | Yes |
| Lipstick Lines | 30-40 years | Atrophy of fat, Pursing muscle of lip, Smoking | Type II | Yes |
| Nasal-labial Fold Lines | 30-40 years | Skin laxity, Pull of smile muscle | Type II | Partial correction |
| Neck Laxity, Early Turkey Wattle | 30-40 years | Skin laxity | Type II | Yes |
| Jowling | 40-50 years | Skin laxity | Type II | Yes |
| Tear Trough Deformity | 50-60 years | Skin laxity, Descent of malar fat pad | Type II | Partial correction |
| Marionette Lines | 50-60 years | Skin laxity, smile muscle pull | Type II | Partial correction |

**TABLE 1-1.**

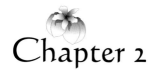

# Chapter 2

# THROUGH
# THE MICROSCOPE

The skin is the body's largest organ, and one of the most important. We cannot live without healthy skin, which is why extensive body burns are so often disabling or fatal. The skin is a living organ, the same as your heart, lungs, liver, stomach and intestines. The skin protects you from the sun and your environment. It holds your vital essence inside. It is the first line of defense against toxins and bacteria. It keeps you hydrated and it plays a crucial role in your immune system, which is your strategic defense system against all foreign invaders. The skin provides wound healing, controls heat loss, produces Vitamin D for your bone health and protects you against some cancers. Skin produces sebum or skin oil which keeps your skin moist, healthy and protected.

# HEALTHY SKIN

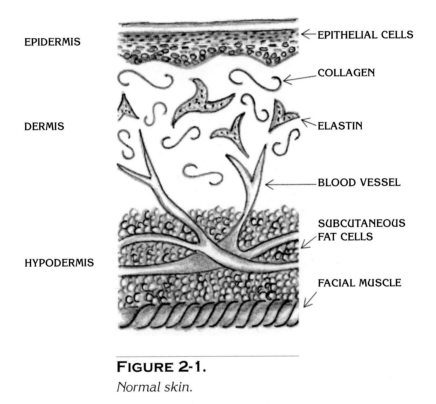

**FIGURE 2-1.**
*Normal skin.*

Let's look through a microscope at a section of healthy, normal, young skin, magnified about 100x. (Figure 2-1).

The outer layer of the skin is the **epidermis**; the cells of the epidermis are called **epithelial cells**. These cells, millions of them, are what you see on the surface of your face. The outer skin surface actually consists of many layers of epithelial cells. New ones are born or formed in the deeper layers every day and then grow upwards to replace the damaged, old, injured cells on the surface.

One reason all anti-aging, beauty, and wrinkle therapies include exfoliation, or removing the top layer of damaged epithelial cells, is that the deeper, newer, plumper, healthier cells look better, and give the skin a fresh glow. It is important to understand that the epithelium is a living layer. As such, it can regenerate, restore and renew itself, which means that you can take steps to prevent and correct aging changes. We'll discuss this more later.

The second, deeper layer of the skin is called the **dermis**. This is where some of the most striking and important changes occur with facial aging, which lead to the loss of elasticity we discussed earlier. That loss of elasticity, you'll recall, is what causes wrinkling and sagging of the face. The dermis is that pink portion of your skin, which you see when you scrape the outer layer of skin. This is the part you see when you injure your knee or hand. It is pink and can bleed when injured deeply. The dermis provides vital life-giving support, oxygen and nutrients to the epidermis. It keeps your outer skin alive. It also provides structural support for your outer skin. It holds your skin onto your body. It helps hold the skin shape.

Three major components of the dermis, which are crucial to the aging process, are: **collagen, elastin** and **hyaluronic acid**. Collagen, a protein, is a major component of the dermis. Collagen is produced by a special cell called the fibroblast. Elastin is a special type of collagen that gives your skin elasticity. Think of elastin as acting like a rubber band that holds your skin on your face. When it is damaged or weakened, your face becomes lax or loose, develops wrinkles and sags.

Hyaluronic acid, known as HA, is a complex substance called a mucopolysaccharide. It is present in the dermis and epidermis. HA surrounds and supports

# SUN DAMAGED SKIN

### ELASTOSIS

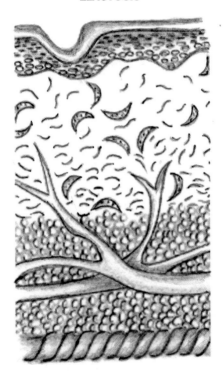

## FIGURE 2-2.

*Sun-damaged skin. The healthy collagen and elastin of the dermis are replaced by fragmented elastin and scar tissue.*

the collagen and all of the cells of the dermis and epidermis. Most importantly, it helps maintain the moisture content of the dermis and the epidermis.

Some of the most striking and important changes that occur with facial aging (and lead to the loss of elasticity and wrinkling we discussed in Chapter One) take place in the dermis. Underneath the dermis is the subcutaneous (under the skin) fat. This supports and protects the skin, nerves, **blood vessels, muscles** and other vital structures. It is a normal component of the skin from the time of birth. **Fat** functions when the skin is bumped, pressed or pushed. Push on the skin of your cheek and notice that the skin virtually slides over the fat, so your skin doesn't tear. Fat also contributes to a healthy skin appearance by its plumping or filling effect. Ever notice how some overweight people do not have wrinkles? So resist the impulse to have your fat sucked out!

Now that you understand the structure of normal healthy skin, let's explore some of the changes that occur as we age and which result in the appearance of the older man shown in the picture in Chapter 1. Look at Figure 2-2, the aged skin, and notice the striking changes. The vital health-sustaining functions of your skin decline to about 1/3 or 2/3 of their normal level by the eighth decade (1). The skin is thinner, due to atrophy (wasting away) of the epidermis, the dermis and the underlying fat. The epidermal cells are less plump and less healthy looking and undergo many changes, which can ultimately lead to skin cancer. Pigment cells increase in an attempt to protect you from the sun, resulting in brown age spots on your face. With thinning of the skin, the blood vessels begin to show through the skin as Telangiectasias or small blood vessels that are most noticeable early around the nose and cheeks. Eventually, the thinning of the skin and the over-growth of blood vessels (caused by free radical damage) produce a pink or red flush on your cheeks and nose, a condition called rosacea. Skin pores are more prominent and large as the supporting collagen around them disappears. These superficial changes are the Type I facial aging changes.

The most striking aging changes take place in the dermis. Over time, collagen and elastin are destroyed and the number of deeper larger blood vessels, oil glands, hair follicles and fibroblasts (recall that they make new collagen) in the dermis decrease.

The dermis thins by 20% as we age (2). The effects of aging are most profound on the type of collagen called elastin, which, you'll recall, is the rubber band-like fiber that holds our skin tight. These fibers are broken, fragmented and lose their ability to give elasticity to our skin. The loss of elasticity allows the skin to sag and wrinkle, while folds form in your face.

The hallmark of sun-damaged, aged skin under the microscope is solar (sun) **elastosis**, seen under the microscope as a large accumulation of damaged elastin piled up in the dermis, replacing the healthy pink collagen seen in normal skin. Remember, this phenomenon causes our facial skin to sag and wrinkle. Almost all modern facial anti-aging treatments – from skinceuticals to lasers, IPL, Thermage®, Titan®, skin peels, and microdermabrasion – attempt to restore new, healthier collagen and will be discussed later.

Hyaluronic acid (HA), the moisturizing matrix supporting your dermis and epidermis is also lost with aging. HA allows nutrients to reach the skin cells. It also holds water, moisturizes the skin, and helps keeps it soft and supple. By age 50, there is a 50% reduction in the HA content of the skin (3). That is huge. No wonder people complain of dry skin at age 50.

In addition, the underlying subcutaneous fat atrophies or wastes away, resulting in loss of its plumping and protective effect on your skin. The muscles beneath your facial skin, which give you facial expression, also ultimately atrophy, but not before they have done their damage. The muscles of facial expression–around your eyes, the smile muscle in the cheek, and those around your mouth – continually contract and pull on your skin throughout your life. The result: Those delightful lines of facial expression, including worry lines, frown lies, bunny lines, crow's feet, smile lines, and lipstick lines. The facial aging changes that occur as a result of these deeper dermal changes are called Type II facial aging changes.

Let's summarize what we have learned in this chapter in the next table (Table 2-1).

| TYPE OF AGING CHANGE | LOCATION OF DAMAGE | WHAT WE SEE |
|---|---|---|
| Type I Aging changes | Epidermis | Dry skin Brown spots Broken blood vessels |
| Type II Aging changes | Dermis Subcutaneous fat | Large pores Wrinkles Skin laxity Lines of facial expression |

**TABLE 2-1.**

# REFERENCES

1. Venna, S.S. and Gilchrest, B.A. Skin aging and photo-aging. Skin & Aging 12:56, 2004

2. Yaar, M. and Gilchrest, B.A. Aging of skin. In I. M. Freidberg, A. Z. Eisen, K. Wolff, et al. (Eds.), Dermatology in General Medicine, New York: McGraw-Hill, 1999. Pp.1697

3. Meschino, J.P. The Wrinkle Free Zone. North Bergen, NJ: Basic Health Publications, 2004. Pp. 49

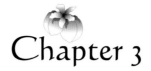

# Chapter 3

# AGING – CELLULAR SUICIDE!

Harsh, but true: We age because the cells that make up our bodies give up and die or are killed by some toxic or harmful thing that we do to them. There are two major types of aging that occur in the cells that make up your face and all of the tissues and organs in your body. The first type is **intrinsic aging**, from the inside. This is a combination of your genetic or inherited aging pattern and your dietary and lifestyle factors, which have a profound influence on the rate and severity of your aging. Second is **extrinsic aging**, (from the outside), referring to the toxic environmental and other harmful factors that damage the health of your skin and accelerate facial aging.

Established science (1, 2) which I believe, tells us that about 80% of skin aging is determined by intrinsic aging and 20% by extrinsic aging. In the sections below we will discuss the specific factors that initiate or cause these harmful aging changes in your skin and your body. I know that this is dry reading, but what you learn here will help you understand what causes facial aging. If you understand what causes facial aging, you can objectively evaluate the proposed cures and decide for yourself if they are realistic and if they make sense to you.

More importantly, the anti-aging therapies we'll discuss will save your face, and they may also save your life. These anti-aging strategies may help you live longer and may lessen your risk for cancer, heart disease, and many other damaging diseases which can end your life prematurely.

Aging is a very complex, multifaceted problem. There is no one theory that is agreed upon by all doctors and scientists. The literature on aging is voluminous, highly technical and hard to understand. Here, I will try to distill a great deal of information in a simplified, comprehensible way which will, I hope, make sense to you and enable you to make some very important decisions about your health. Be patient and read on.

# INTRINSIC AGING
# THE CELL — THE BASIC BUILDING
# BLOCK OF LIFE

Our bodies are made up of billions of tiny cells. In Chapter 2, you saw pictures of the cells that make up the outer layer of our skin, the epithelial cells. Every structure in our body is made up of specialized cells–our muscles, bones, brain, gut, liver, and all of our life giving tissues. When enough of these cells die, we die! A heart attack kills the cells of the heart, so that the heart can no longer function to pump blood to our brain and body and we die. Some of our body parts are more important than others. We can live after losing a leg or an eye, but not without a functioning heart.

When we are born, if we do not have a birth defect, the cells of our body are healthy and function properly, a state we call good health [Figure 3-1]. To stay healthy and grow each of our cells must be able to divide into two new cells, over and over again. This is a very vital process by which we grow into adulthood and by which we maintain our health. After we become adults,

# HEALTHY CELL

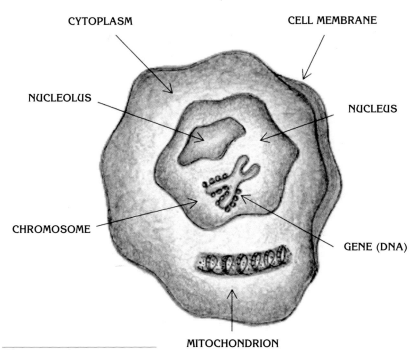

**FIGURE 3-1.**

*Healthy cell, the basic structural unit of all life.*

the daily work of living, digesting food, resisting infection, walking, working – virtually everything we do – requires the cells of our body to work very hard to keep us alive. Eventually our cells wear out, so the old cells must divide to create new cells, so that our bodies continue to function.

However, our cells cannot go on dividing forever. In fact, most cells are programmed at birth to divide only 70 times during the course of one's life (3). Eventually they stop dividing and die and no new cells are produced. When enough of our vital, life-sustaining cells no longer function, we die. Cell death is, in essence, intrinsic aging.

Why does this happen to our cells? Why can't they divide forever and allow us to go on living forever? It is God's will, perhaps. Theorists opine that once we have passed our childbearing years we have outlived our usefulness to the planet, since our essential role is to produce offspring and renew life on the earth. Once this task is accomplished, this line of thinking supports that we must age and die so there will be adequate resources such as food and space for new generations of humans.

Another important reason that our cells are not allowed to divide indefinitely and uncontrollably, is that uncontrolled cell division is cancer. A cancer is basically a mass of uncontrollable, rapidly dividing cells.

Uncontrolled dividing of breast cells is breast cancer. Uncontrolled dividing of colon cells is colon cancer, and so on. Thus, our bodies must be able to control cell division or we could develop cancer in any of our body organs. The key to discovering a cure for cancer is discovering how to turn off the uncontrolled cell division and thus, kill the cancer by making it grow old.

## INSIDE YOUR CELLS – DNA AND YOUR GENETIC HERITAGE

DNA is a protein that makes up our genes, tiny packets of information that are attached to our chromosomes (Figure 3-2).

Chromosomes reside in the center of our cells in the nucleus. Every time our cells divide, the chromosomes divide, carrying a complete set of genes and DNA to each of the two new cells. The DNA present in your genes spells out specific messages or detailed instructions to your cells to tell them what to do, what to make and when to divide.

## HEALTHY CHROMOSOME

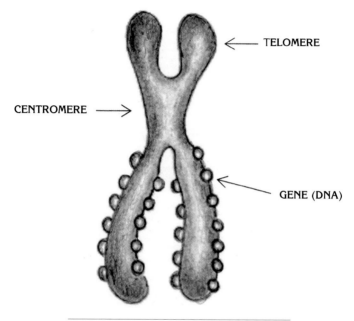

**FIGURE 3-2.**
*Healthy chromosome with attached genes consisting of DNA.*

DNA is the basic structure that controls all of the functions of every cell in our bodies. Thus, our DNA is the ultimate factor that determines when and how we age. Have you noticed how some people look young for their age? I have seen people in their 50s who look like they are 30 years old, and I am a professional at evaluating facial aging! Other 40-year-old people have gray hair, deep wrinkles, and sagging skin, while another person the same age has dark hair and smooth moist skin, with no wrinkles or laxity. The difference between these individuals is due to the difference in their DNA. (Some would call it luck!)

There are six basic types of skin and each one is determined by heredity. See Table 3-1 below and identify your skin type.

| Skin, Hair & Eye Color | Skin Type | Tendency to Burn | Tendency to Tan | Tendency to Age | Type of Aging Changes |
|---|---|---|---|---|---|
| White- red- blue | Type I | Always | Never | Early & severe | Type I & II |
| White- blond- blue or brown | Type II | Usually | Sometimes | Early | Type I & II |
| White- brown- dark- brown | Type III | Usually | Usually | Later | Type II |
| Brown to black- black- brown | Type IV-VI | Never | Always | Very late | Type II |

**TABLE 3-1.**
*Hereditary skin types.*

The information that controls the type of skin we have is carried in the DNA in our genes on the chromosomes that we inherit from our parents.

Understanding your skin type is important because different skin types age very differently. Your inherited DNA, plus your nutrition, lifestyle, and exposure to toxins, not only determines how you look and how your skin ages but also how the rest of your body ages. We now know that heart disease, cancer, and many of the diseases that lead to premature aging, disability and death are influenced by our heredity. But do not despair: We now can do a great deal to forestall or prevent these genetic catastrophes by lifestyle and nutritional modifications (see Chapter 4). The ultimate goal of the Human Genome Project is to figure out how to modify genes to stop or prevent diseases that cause human suffering, disease, and death. If you want to learn more about genes and chromosomes, visit http://encarta.msn.com/enc-net/refpages/RefArticle.aspxefid=761566230&pn=1 &s=2.

## THE TELOMERE —
## YOUR BIOLOGICAL AGING CLOCK

A **telomere** is a small DNA tail attached to each of your chromosomes (Figure 3-2). The telomere protects your chromosomes during cell division. When cells divide, they do so only after the chromosomes divide and it is important that each new cell has all the genes necessary to be a healthy, functioning cell. There is a risk that, during the cell division process, the chromosomes can be damaged and lose some of the genes. If genes and the crucial DNA they contain are lost, the new cells cannot function normally and can die or, worse, create abnormal products that can cause harm. The telomere protects the end of the chromosome by keeping it together, preventing the loss of any genes during the division of the chromosome. This is a very important function.

As we age and as our cells keep dividing, the telomere loses some of its DNA each time the cell divides, and the telomere keeps getting shorter. Some scientists theorize that when our telomeres are shortened too much or are lost, the cells die–and so do we. Research has also associated short telomeres in people with short life spans, but some animals with longer telomeres than humans have shorter life spans than humans, so we do not have all the answers yet.

Scientists have discovered an enzyme called telomerase, which can prevent telomeres from getting shorter when the cell divides. Researchers theorize that if telomerase can be used to prevent shortening of the telomere, cell division can go on indefinitely and therefore we, and our cells, can become immortal. The problem is, unrestrained or immortal cell division is cancer and in fact telomerase may well play a role in cancer cell growth. Some scientists hope that blocking telomerase may be a way to kill cancer cells and cure cancer. This field is very exciting and future discoveries will undoubtedly impact both cancer and aging research. If you want to read more information on telomeres, visit http://gslc.genetics.utah.edu/features/telomeres/.

# FREE RADICALS DESTROY OUR CELLS AND DNA, CAUSE INFLAMMATION, AND CAUSE FACIAL AGING

If you have not heard about free radicals by now, you certainly will very soon. Chances are, if you purchased this book, you already pop a mouthful of antioxidant vitamins every morning. If you do, swell, you are halfway there. Free radicals have a major impact on facial aging and this topic is so important and the discovery of new relevant therapies is occurring so rapidly, that I think it is important for you to have a good understanding of this subject.

Let's re-visit Biology 101 for a moment. The cells in our bodies are made up of complex molecules, and molecules are made up of atoms. The atom, the basic submicroscopic unit of which we are made, has positive (+) electrical charges called protons (+) on the inside and negative (-) electrical charges called electrons (-) on the outside. The electrons spin around the protons in the center of the atom like a satellite spins around the earth, being held in orbit by the gravitational pull of the earth.

The electrons which have a negative charge (-) are kept close to the atom by the pull of the opposite, positive (+) charge of the protons. This is similar to the way opposite ends of two magnets are attracted and attach to each other (Figure 3-3).

## STABLE ATOM

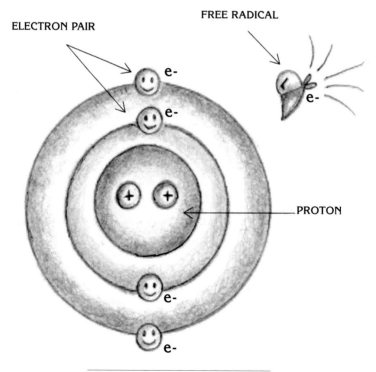

**FIGURE 3-3.**
*An atom with stable electrons in orbit.*

The two opposite charges together are in balance and exert no charge or effect on the rest of the cell. The electrons that exert one negative (-) charge actually consist of two small spinning electrons, which, together, represent one negative (-) charge. There is a lot of energy holding the electron pair in the orbit around the proton in the center of the atom. These paired charges, that is the proton (+) and electron pair (-), keep the atom stable, like a good marriage (Figure 3-3).

A free radical is formed when some outside force steals or knocks one of the paired electrons away from its stable orbit around the atom (Figure 3-4). The result? The atom that has lost the electron becomes very unstable. It now has an unpaired electron in the outer orbit, so it is now a free radical. It creates havoc in your cells by searching around and trying to steal a negatively charged electron (-) away from another stable atom that has paired electrons in the outer orbit. The free radical scientists (in reality most of them are very tame, but they like the name) often call these free radicals "promiscuous" (are the scientists projecting?)

# UNSTABLE ATOM

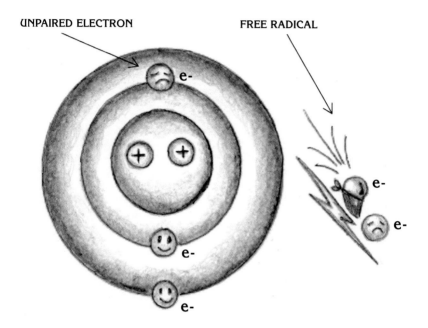

UNSTABLE ATOM NOW BECOMES A FREE RADICAL

## FIGURE 3-4.
*A free radical is formed.*

These "promiscuous" free radicals scurry around your cells and create intracellular havoc. On a cellular level this is a very high energy-process not unlike a hurricane or an earthquake is to us. A lot of damage is produced in your cells when free radicals are

# UNHEALTHY CELL

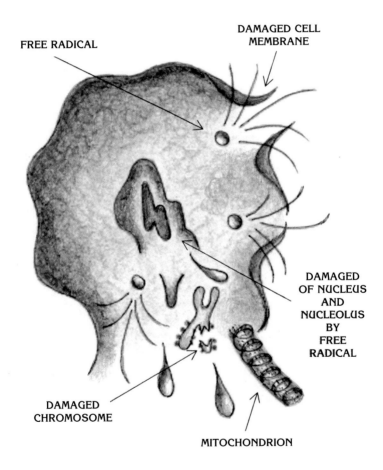

**FIGURE 3-5.**

*Free radicals damage cell wall
and DNA (genes) on chromosome.*

formed. How does this process damage your cells? In two ways:

First, free radicals damage your cell membrane, the essential shell that keeps the contents of your cell inside. This damage can kill the cell or, if the damage is not fatal, it impacts the ability of your cell to carry out important life-sustaining functions (Figure 3-5). Second, when free radicals attack, they damage your DNA. This can destroy the genes that control your cells' vital functions (Figure 3-6).

Where do free radicals come from? Believe it or not, most of the free radicals in our bodies come from the oxygen we breathe. Oxygen is used by the **mito-chondria**, which are small structures in our cells that convert our food into energy (Figure 3-7). During this process, a great number of free radicals are produced (Figure3-8).

Fortunately, our bodies have built-in protective mechanisms called free radical scavengers that clean up these free radicals before they can do harm.

# UNHEALTHY CHROMOSOME

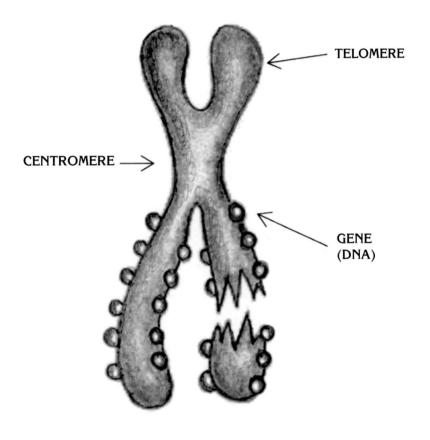

**FIGURE 3-6.**

*Chromosome with damage by
free radicals.*

# HEALTHY MITOCHONDRION

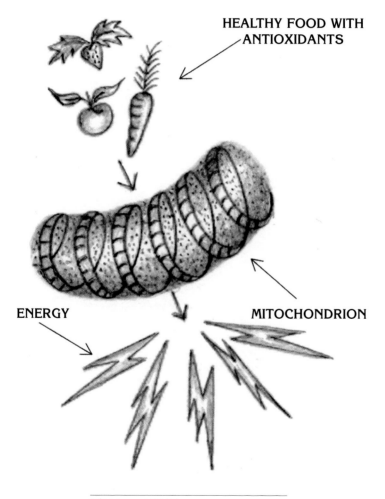

HEALTHY FOOD WITH ANTIOXIDANTS

ENERGY

MITOCHONDRION

## FIGURE 3-7.

*Healthy mitochondria in the cell convert our food to energy.*

# UNHEALTHY MITOCHONDRION

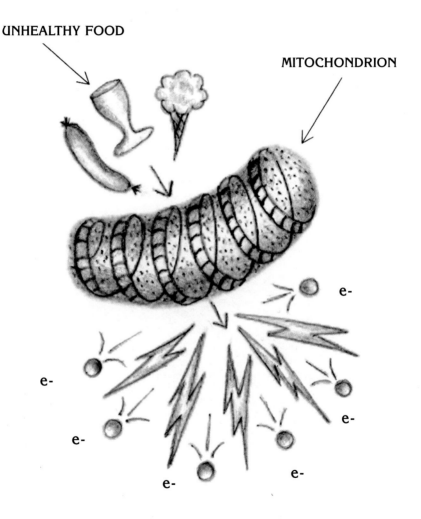

**UNHEALTHY FOOD**

**MITOCHONDRION**

e-

e-

e-

e-

e-

e-

## FIGURE 3-8.

*Mitochondria also produce free radicals during the energy production process, especially when unhealthy foods are ingested.*

The free radical scavengers require the presence of the antioxidant vitamins C, A, and E (and many others) in proper amounts for this protective system to work. When we do not have adequate amounts of these important vitamins or we are subjected to too many free radicals, the system is overloaded, damage occurs, and our cells are either destroyed or no longer function normally.

In summary, free radicals are formed as follows:

- We eat food.
- Food is broken down and the nutrients go into our cells and into the mitochondria.
- The mitochondria take the food, add oxygen and make energy to keep us alive.
- Energy production produces atoms with good, paired electrons, but also produces some free radicals.

These free radicals damage the cell membrane and DNA. The end result: Your cells die or are altered in such a way that they produce very harmful products (4).

# INFLAMMATION – THE BASIC CAUSE OF FACIAL AGING

When our DNA and cell membranes are injured by free radicals (or anything else for that matter), the damaged cell membrane releases a toxic substance called **arachidonic acid**. The damaged DNA also causes the release of **cytokines**, the chemical messengers that tell the rest of the body that damage has occurred. Both of these substances initiate a process called inflammation.

Inflammation is the response of the cells of our body to injury, cell damage or death. This damage can be caused by trauma, toxins, bacteria, viruses or other foreign invaders as well as by free radicals. Inflammation is the attempt by our body to stop and isolate the damage and keep it from spreading.

The signals put out by the damaged cells, carried by cytokines, tell our blood to send in **macrophages**. These are specialized blood cells that actually eat the damaged cells and remove them from the area. The macrophages then take the damaged cells back to the blood stream and eventually to our lymph nodes, from which they are removed from the body. Inflammation is a very important life-saving process. It protects us from harmful bacterial infection. It helps heal our wounds, and removes dead or damaged cells from our bodies.

The problem is, inflammation also produces some damaging chemicals and events inside our bodies which contribute to facial aging. Worse, inflammation can be turned against us in a way that results in an autoimmune response. An autoimmune response occurs when inflammation attacks and destroys our own normal body cells. This is disastrous, and scientists are discovering that many of the diseases we attribute to old age, such as heart disease, some cancers, and Alzheimer's disease, may in fact be caused by our own inflammatory processes turned against us.

Inflammation initiates a series of chain reactions when started by the cytokines. The macrophages not only clean up the damaged cells, they also send messages to bring other cells called **mast cells** to release **histamine**, a substance which dilates your blood vessels. Histamine makes the blood vessels leaky, and the injured site becomes filled with fluid and blood. This is why an injured site on the body turns red and is swollen. One very relevant example of inflammation with regard to facial aging is the sunburn.

Prolonged or severe inflammation is very destructive to the cells and tissues that the body is trying to protect and heal. Once the dead cells and debris are cleaned up, the macrophages convert to fibroblasts, which, you'll recall, are the cells that produce collagen. The collagen produced during inflammation is a scar. When free radicals cause damage to your cells and produce inflammation in your skin, your healthy collagen is destroyed, and the scar collagen functions poorly. The result is wrinkles and damaged, sagging skin.

# Hormones — Internal Modulators of Cell Function

Hormones are substances secreted by the glands of our body: the pituitary gland in the brain, the thyroid gland in our neck, the pancreas near our stomach, and the adrenal gland which sits atop our kidneys. These hormones serve vital, life – giving roles by stimulating the cells of our body to carry out the important functions that keep us alive. As we age, the levels of various hormones decline and cellular functions dependent on these hormones also decline. These events have a major impact on facial aging.

It is important to understand that hormone replacement therapies should be used only when clinically significant deficiencies exist. Notice I said when deficiencies exist. Hormone replacement should only be done with a doctor's supervision.

# Cortisol — The Stress Hormone

Elevated levels of the adrenal hormone **cortisol** have a dramatic and profound aging effect on the cells of our face and body. When you are stressed, you worry, and we have already discussed the damaging effects of the worry lines on your face. More importantly, cortisol is very damaging to the cells that make up your facial skin and other important organs in your body. Cortisol is a hormone released by your adrenal glands when you are in danger and need to go on "high alert" to protect yourself. Cortisol speeds up your heart, pushes blood into your muscles, increases the energy produced by your muscle cells, and basically prepares you for "fight or flight." The problem is that if you stay pumped up like this all the time, you exhaust the cells of your body

The stress of living in contemporary society, where we overextend ourselves and live under immense time pressure, causes our adrenal glands to produce excess cortisol. Prolonged, excessively high cortisol levels worsen intrinsic facial aging changes by directly damaging collagen. It disturbs the pancreatic hormone insulin's ability to properly metabolize sugar and fats, and can deplete the body's immune system, all of which can lead to inflammation (3).

# ESTROGEN, PROGESTERONE AND TESTOSTERONE — THE SEX HORMONES

The sex hormones have profound effects on facial aging. During menopause, there is a 90% decrease in estrogen levels and a 66% decrease in progesterone, both of which cause thinning and dryness of the skin (5). In male andropause, testosterone levels drop by 50% (6), which, not only thins the skin but also, reduces muscle mass.

# HUMAN GROWTH HORMONE (HGH)

Produced by the pituitary gland, HGH also decreases during aging. Replacement therapy has been associated with restoration of muscle mass, energy, libido, and improvement in skin aging changes–hooray! However, the only proven regimen that works is by injection. Most oral forms, which are supposed to stimulate your pituitary gland to make more HGH, do not work.

More importantly, I'm afraid to take HGH injections for a very key reason: HGH works by making cells in your body divide to make brand – new cells. Remember, cells dividing too much also cause cancer. Intelligent medical opinion holds that not enough is known about HGH cell-dividing stimulation to be sure that it is safe. Have your doctor check your HGH level. If it is low, consider replacement therapy. If it is normal, then I recommend not taking HGH. Personally, I would rather have wrinkles than cancer any day.

## MELATONIN – THE ANTI-AGING HORMONE

Melatonin, a hormone secreted by the pineal gland in your brain, is called the anti-aging hormone. It is a powerful antioxidant and free radical scavenger and is also reported to play a role in supporting our immune system and thus fighting inflammation (7, 8). It also plays an important role in our sleep/wake cycles, which enable us to rest and our body to restore itself. Melatonin is depleted by the stress hormone cortisol.

# Extrinsic Aging

Traditionally, a discussion of extrinsic aging focused only on the damage caused by UV (ultraviolet) light from the rays of the sun on the skin. However, as our knowledge of the aging process has expanded, we have become aware of a host of other things that we take into our bodies that also cause significant free radical damage and contribute to the aging process. I'm including some of these factors in the extrinsic aging category because we choose whether or not we take them into our bodies.

# Sunlight

The ultraviolet (UV) wavelengths of the sun's rays have a dramatic, destructive aging effect on your skin, especially if you are a fair-skinned Type I or Type II skin type. UV radiation damages the epithelial cells and destroys your collagen and elastin and is a major cause of the Type I skin changes discussed in Chapter 2. There is much evidence that the aging effect of the sun directly causes cellular damage and also produces free radicals, which damage the cell walls and DNA of the skin cells (9). If you want a graphic example of the aging effects of the sun on your skin, compare the skin of your face to that of your underarm.

## ENVIRONMENTAL TOXINS

There are many other environmental toxins that contribute to the aging process. Tobacco smoke has a profound aging effect on the skin – not to mention your lungs, heart, and blood vessels – most likely by producing free radicals. Other environmental pollutants believed to contribute to the free radical load imposed on your body include:

- Pesticides
- X-rays
- Drugs
- Exhaust fumes

## THE FOOD WE EAT

The modern diet, so heavily dependent on processed foods, is sorely lacking in the necessary antioxidant vitamins and minerals necessary for healthy cellular function and protection from free radical damage. Worse, our high consumption of refined starches, sugars, saturated fats, and animal fat actually produces free radicals and add a significant burden of free radicals to our already nutritionally depleted body cells. An in-depth discussion of this topic is beyond the scope of this book. To read more about the nutritional aspects of aging, check out the excellent book by Dr. Vincent Giampappa et al. (3). The following are dietary products that contribute to facial aging:

- Sugar
- Alcohol
- Highly processed starches (potato chips etc.)
- Animal fats
- BBQ and smoked meats
- Nitrate or nitrite-containing foods (such as bacon)
- Charred meat and fish

Let's summarize what we have learned about the many controllable factors that contribute to the aging process and cause the dramatic and disheartening changes we see in our faces as we age in Table 3-2.

| AGING FACTOR | INTRINSIC | EXTRINSIC | SOURCE | HOW TO PREVENT |
|---|---|---|---|---|
| Heredity | X | | Genes DNA | Human Genome Project |
| Free Radicals | X | X | Environment Diet Our own cells | Diet Vitamins Lifestyle modification |
| Inflammation | X | X | Environment Diet Lifestyle | Diet Vitamins Lifestyle modification |
| Cortisol | X | | Stress | Lifestyle modification |
| Estrogen | X | | Ovaries | Diet Supplements Vitamins |
| Progesterone | X | | Ovaries | Diet Supplements Vitamins |
| Testosterone | X | | Testes | Diet Supplements Vitamins Replacement |

**TABLE 3-2.**

| AGING FACTOR | INTRINSIC | EXTRINSIC | SOURCE | HOW TO PREVENT |
|---|---|---|---|---|
| Human Growth Hormone (HGH) | X | | Pituitary Gland | Replacement |
| Melatonin | X | | Pineal Gland | Replacement |
| Sunlight – UV radiation | | X | The Sun | Avoid sun Sun protection |
| Toxins – tobacco, x-rays, pesticides etc | | X | Environmental Lifestyle | Avoid |
| Dietary – alcohol, refined sugars and starches, animal and saturated fats | | X | Diet | Avoid |

**TABLE 3-2. CONTINUED**

The good news is that out of the 12 major causes of intrinsic aging, you can take definitive action to reverse or prevent 11 of them! That is very exciting news and should really motivate you to study the next chapter on prevention. Furthermore, with the exciting progress being made by the Human Genome Project, someday, in the not too distant future, we will be able to modify our genes to slow the aging process.

Well, my cortisol levels are so high after 12 hours at the computer that my melatonin levels are getting dangerously low. I can feel the free radicals trying to initiate the inflammatory cascade in my neck and shoulders, and if I am not careful I won't be able to do any book signings. So I am going to go to sleep and let my pineal gland do its thing!

## REFERENCES

1.  Venna, S.S. and Gilchrest, B.A. Skin aging and photo-aging. Skin & Aging 12:56, 2004

2.  El-Domyati, M., Attia, S., Saleh, F., et al. Intrinsic aging vs. photo-aging: a comparative histopathological, immunohistochemical, and ultrastructural study of skin. Exper. Dermatol. 11:398, 2002

3.  Giampapa, V., Pero, R., and Zimmerman, M. The Anti-aging Solution. Hoboken: Wiley, 2004 Pp. 20 and Pp.43-45

4.  Proctor, P. H. Free radicals and Human disease. CRC Handbook of Free Radicals and Antioxidants. 1: 209, 1989.

5.  Meschino, J.P. The Wrinkle Free Zone. North Bergen, NJ: Basic Health Publications, 2004. Pp. 94.

6.  Klatz, R., and Goldman, R. Stopping the Clock-Longevity for the New Millenniun, 2nd ED. North Berg, New Jersy: Basic Health publications, 2002. Pp. 47.

7. Armstrong, S.M., and Redman, J.R. Melatonin: a chronobiotic with anti-aging properties? Med. Hypotheses. 34: 300-309, 1991

8. Pierpaoli, W. and Changxian, Y. The involvement of pineal gland and melatonin in immunity and aging. J. Neuroimmunol. 27:99-109, 1990.

9. Nishigori, C., Hattori, Y., Arima, Y., et al. Photo-aging and oxidative stress. Exper. Dermatol. 12(suppl. 2): 18-21, 2003

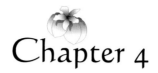

# Chapter 4

# How to Save Your Face — Feed Your Mind, Body, and Spirit

There is a major and exciting revolution in health care occurring today and you are the main beneficiary! I am talking about the anti-aging revolution, which started many years ago. It began quietly, with a few bright, devoted scientists who knew in their hearts that nature held the key to disease prevention, cure, and longevity. Without science to back them up, they have been viewed with suspicion by traditional organized medicine, and labeled "Alternative Medicine." But science has finally caught up with the early visionaries and today we can talk seriously about effective anti-aging strategies and realistically start taking steps to stop and reverse the aging of your face and your body.

The birth of HMOs, (health maintenance organizations), was a great concept, designed to reduce health care costs by preventing disease, but it has failed miserably. Instead of promoting health by prevention, the HMOs have simply attempted, unsuccessfully, to reduce health care costs by rationing health care to you, the patient, and cutting payments to hospitals and doctors. No wonder so many hospitals have closed, and no wonder that when you call for help, you are likely to get an answering machine instead of a doctor!

Thank God for the "Alternative Medicine" movement! As my father always said, "If you want something done right, do it yourself." This adage has never been truer than it is today with regard to your health. That is why you bought this book and that is why our generation is taking action and being responsible for our own health

Fortunately, you already know about the damage free radicals can do to you and you are taking action. It will be worth your while. Our generation is accustomed to taking the lead and not blindly accepting the status quo. Your health is the most important cause you can support.

The truth in facial aging is the same as the truth in every human disease: Prevention is the best cure, or, as the saying goes, "an ounce of prevention is worth a pound of cure." Nowhere is that principle more evident or easier to apply than on the facial skin, our most visible and accessible body part. So let's learn what we can do to protect ourselves and prevent facial aging.

## ANTI-AGING THERAPY

### Sun Block Can Save Your Life!

Sunlight not only ages you, it can kill you, no matter what the color of your skin. Skin damage by the ultraviolet (UV) rays of the sun is one of the most important extrinsic causes of facial aging. More importantly, UV light from the sun causes skin cancers: basal cell carcinoma, squamous cell carcinoma and melanoma. The following statistics should horrify you into taking action:

Invasive melanoma is a highly malignant, often fatal type of skin cancer. In 1935, Americans had a 1 in 1500 risk of developing invasive melanoma in their lifetime. This rate increased to 1 in 250 by 1980 and to 1 in 74 by 2001 and it is estimated that it will be 1 in 50 by the year 2010 (1). Increased sun exposure due to increased outdoor activities, tanning booths, and more revealing clothing undoubtedly play a part in this virtual epidemic. Loss of the protective ozone layer may be another important cause. A frightening fact is that 10% of US teenagers use tanning booths and two thirds don't apply sunscreens when outdoors (2). One third of adults in one study admitted to having suffered sunburn in the previous year (2). The important point is that sun protection is the most important yet most often neglected anti-aging and cancer preventing treatment you can use.

Sun block alone is not enough. New research indicates that the addition of topical antioxidant vitamins C, A, E, and melatonin (3, 4, 5) significantly increase protection from the harmful effects of sunlight above and beyond the protection afforded by sun block alone. The newer sun blocks contain the antioxidant vitamins A, C, E, and others (Figure 4-1). When you are outside, exposed to the sun:

- Wear a wide-brimmed hat. You must protect the ears, as well as the face.
- Wear UV protecting wrap-around sunglasses and sun-protective clothing, such as wet suits or "rash guards" for your children.

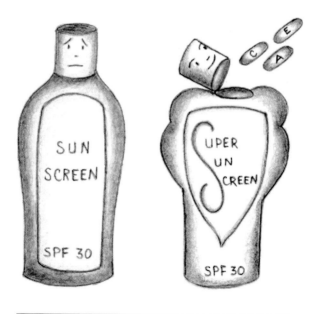

**FIGURE 4-1.**

*Newer sunscreens containing antioxidant vitamins are more effective.*

- Stay out of the sun during the peak hours, 10 a.m. to 2 p.m.
- Apply an even coating of sun block using 30 grams or one ounce for the whole body. Apply at least 30 minutes before going into the sun.
- Reapply sun block regularly every one to two hours, at minimum. Be certain to cover the area around your eyes, nose, lips, and ears, the parts of your face that get the most sun, but are often missed.
- A sun block with a SPF 15, antioxidant vitamins and one that also blocks both UVA and UVB is a minimum. Children and adults with Type I skin (redheads) and Type II skin (fair skinned blue eyed blondes) who have high sun exposure should wear a minimum of SPF 30.
- Follow the guidelines, even on cloudy days. 80% of UV rays are transmitted even on a cloudy day.
- Total protection for your children is even more important because up to 80% of sun exposure occurs during childhood.
- Teach your children the Australian saying SLIP, SLOP, SLAP AND WRAP – "Slip on a shirt, slop on sunscreen, slap on a hat and wrap-around sunglasses"

# Antioxidants and Nutritional Supplements Prevent Cellular Suicide

Our skin is a vibrant, living organ, the largest organ of our bodies. In Chapter 3, you learned how free radical damage occurring in our cells causes aging, cell death and cancer. Fortunately, nature has provided us with natural antioxidant vitamins and minerals that work inside our cells to neutralize the damaging free radicals and make them harmless. This process is called scavenging and the vitamins and minerals that remove free radicals are called free radical scavengers.

It is essential that we have adequate levels of these free radical scavengers present in our cells. The way nature intended for us to get these important vitamins and minerals was through our diet. Long ago, when we were "cave men and women," we survived on the fruits, nuts and berries provided by nature and the occasional meat we were lucky enough to obtain through hunting or scavenging the kills of larger animals, or animals that died of injury or disease. This early diet, primarily consisting of fruits and vegetables, was rich in antioxidant vitamins and minerals, complex carbohydrates, and proteins, and low in fat. Obviously, this diet allowed our species to flourish and populate the earth! In these earlier times people rarely lived long enough to develop chronic diseases such as diabetes, heart disease, and arthritis. Early humans were killed off at an early age – certainly before their thirties – by accident, bigger animals, or infections, but not by old age.

As humans learned to control the supply of food necessary to survive by domesticating animals and farming, our diet began to change. We learned how to process or refine starches and sugars, creating white bread from wheat, and white crystallized sugar from natural sugar. We learned to domesticate and fatten livestock for a steady supply of meat high in fat content. These developments and the discovery of antibiotics to treat infections increased the human lifespan to the seventies. However, our new modern diet also set the stage for the development of many modern-day diseases such as diabetes, obesity, heart disease, and cancer.

The processing, refining, and preservation of much of our food supply removes the essential antioxidants that nature has provided for us in the fruits and vegetables that were a dietary staple millions of years ago. Worse, much of what we eat, especially fat, actually contains or creates more free radicals than the free radical scavenger systems of our body can handle. So, you might say, what we eat is actually killing us!

As a result, it is necessary to add antioxidant vitamins and minerals and foods high in antioxidants to our diet if we want to prevent or reverse some of the free radical mediated damage to our facial skin. The following is a brief discussion of many of the antioxidant vitamins minerals, and compounds, and the recommended daily dosages.

## VITAMIN A

Vitamin A and its precursor, beta-carotene, are found in yellow, green and orange vegetables, egg yolks, liver, butter and fish oils. Vitamin A and the derivatives of vitamin A are called the **retinoids**, which are an important ingredient in many skin medications. Retinoids regulate the growth of the epidermal cells, inhibit the formation of cancer, decrease inflammation and improve immune function in the skin (6, 7). Vitamin A and its derivatives are powerful antioxidants, and studies have shown that this compound can decrease and reverse the signs of aging of the skin (7). Current recommendations for supplementation are Vitamin A 2500 IU or Beta Carotene the Vitamin A precursor 10,000 IU/day.

Vitamin A and its derivatives can cause birth defects, and excessive doses can cause increased pressure on your brain. Therefore, Vitamin A and beta-carotene should not be taken by women who are pregnant and dosages higher than those recommended should be avoided.

## VITAMIN C

Vitamin C is a powerful antioxidant and is also important in new collagen formation, wound healing and the formation of the prostaglandin hormones

PG1 and PG3, substances that play an important role in making the skin smooth and soft. Vitamin C plays an important role in the regeneration of Vitamin E. Vitamin C has also been shown to enhance the protection of your skin from the harmful effects of UV radiation from sunlight! (7, 8). Daily dosage is 1000 mg.

## VITAMIN E

Vitamin E is a fat-soluble vitamin, found in your cell membranes. It is an important free radical scavenger that works to prevent damage to the cell membrane, which, you'll recall, is one of the vital structures to which free radicals produce their most damaging effects on your cells. Clinically, Vitamin E has been shown to have beneficial effects on LDL cholesterol, heart disease, and immune function (9). Daily dose is 400 IU.

Vitamin E can interfere with the ability of your blood to clot, so do not take this vitamin if you are on coumadin or other blood thinners.

## SELENIUM

Selenium is a mineral that acts as a beneficial antioxidant in cholesterol metabolism. It has been shown to have beneficial effects on heart disease, cancer, and the immune system. Levels of this mineral in our body drop 7 to 24% by age 70 (10). Selenium is found in Brazil nuts, sunflower seeds, grains, meat, garlic, and seafood. It plays an important role in the antioxidant protection of the skin. Recommended dosage is 70 mcg. daily.

## ZINC

Zinc is necessary for the production of superoxide dismutase, an important antioxidant enzyme. It plays an important role in immunity and wound healing. Recommended dosage is 30-50 mg. daily (11).

## MAGNESIUM

Magnesium participates in antioxidant activity that protects cell membranes and the mitochondria. It is also is very important in regulating calcium balance. It is found in whole grains, nuts, seeds and legumes. Recommended daily dose is 400mg. daily (12).

## COENZYME Q10

Coenzyme Q10 is necessary for the production of enzyme Q10 in the mitochondria in your cells. It also acts as an antioxidant, protecting the cell membrane. (13). Recently, Coenzyme Q10 has been used to reverse congestive heart failure (14). However, there have also been controlled clinical studies which failed to show a beneficial effect of Coenzyme Q10 in heart disease (15).

The statin drugs used to lower cholesterol can deplete Coenzyme Q10 (16). Recommended dose is 30 to 280 mg. daily. However, this drug can interact with many other drugs, so you should consult your doctor before taking Coenzyme Q10.

## ALPHA LIPOIC ACID – ALA

Alpha Lipoic acid is important in the regeneration of the antioxidants Vitamin C, Vitamin E, and Coenzyme Q10, and helps protect DNA from metals that can generate free radicals (17). ALA can also help prevent glycation, the harmful effect of sugar in the blood. Recommended dose is 100mg per day (18).

## L-CARNITINE

L-Carnitine assists in the transport of fats across the cell membrane and thus assists in the burning of fats for energy production. It is also important in enhancing the effects of Coenzyme Q10. Recommended supplement is 50-100mg per day (19).

## SULFUR-CONTAINING ANTIOXIDANTS

Sulfur containing vegetables such as cruciferous vegetables, and garlic have antioxidant properties and are important for immune function. Recommended dosage is extract of cruciferous vegetables 500-1000mg, and Garlic 100mg per day (20).

## Repair Your DNA-CAE's

In Chapter 3, we discussed the crucial role of DNA damage in the aging process. There is exciting new evidence that it may be possible to reverse DNA damage. Dr. Ron Pero, a molecular biologist in Lund, Sweden, has isolated a group of compounds called carboxy alkyl esters (CAE's ) which he purports actually stimulate DNA repair enzymes when paired with nicotinamide (a B vitamin ), zinc, and natural carotines. The author cites studies which show these compounds can improve immunity and decrease inflammation. He recommends CAE extract 350mg per day taken with Medicinal mushroom extracts 500-100mg per day (21).

## Fatty Acid Supplements

While most animal fats are harmful, the fatty acids known as Omega-3 oils have many health positive benefits. Remember how the cell wall contains fats and fats play an essential role in protecting your skin? Cold-water fish and dark green vegetables are natural sources of good fatty acids. Dr Giampappa (22) recommends Fish omega – 3 blend of EPA-300mg, DHA-500mg, 1000-3000 mg per day.

## B VITAMINS

B vitamins play an important role in skin health. Deficiency syndromes include cracks in the lips (Riboflavin B-2 deficiency), pellagra – a condition causing a rash and rough skin (Niacin B-3 deficiency), and skin pigmentation (vitamin B12 deficiency). Vitamin B5, also known as panthenol the active form of panthothenic acid, is widely used as a humectant or moisturizer for the skin. Vitamin B3 and B6 also play a role in Prostaglandin (PG) synthesis which helps maintain skin softness. The B vitamins are playing an important role in cellular energy production, protection of DNA, and in the proper function of your genes. A B-50 complex vitamin daily is recommended for optimal skin health (23).

# Prostaglandin Hormones (PG)

Prostaglandin hormones (PG) are made by skin cells from fats in the diet. PG1 and PG3 work together to moisten the skin and make it soft. They are not to be confused with Prostaglandins 2 (PG2), which are harmful byproducts of the oxidation product arachidonic acid. According to Dr. Meschino (24), PG1 synthesis is optimized by supplementation with Borage oil and PG3 synthesis is enhanced by supplementing with fish oil and flaxseed oil. He recommends the following:

- Reduce intake of high fat meats and dairy products which increase PG2 synthesis.
- Substitute olive oil, canola oil, and/or peanut oil in place of corn, sunflower, safflower seed and mixed vegetable oils.

# Detoxification – Remove Skin Damaging Toxins From Your Body

Our liver is the primary organ in our body responsible for detoxifying, that is making harmless, dangerous substances that have accumulated in our blood. The liver detoxifies excess hormones our body produces and other chemicals we produce internally. The liver also detoxifies medications, alcohol, pesticides and other environmental contaminants. As we age, our liver detoxification system can slow down due to the accumulation of toxic substances, for instance alcohol, age or other damage such as hepatitis. Failure of liver detoxification can allow harmful toxic substances to build up in our blood, many of which are Free Radicals and can increase skin aging changes. Dr. Meshino (25) recommends a daily detoxification protocol for optimum skin health and anti-aging nutritional support. His recommendations are listed in the protocol below:

## DETOXIFICATION PROTOCOL

- Cruciferous vegetables (broccoli)
- Grapefruit, Oranges
- Soy extract
- Milk Thistle 150-600mg
- Vitamin C 1000 mg

- Indole-3 Carbinol 25-100mg
- Reischi Mushroom Extract – 30 mg to 120 mg
- Astragalus 100 mg to 400mg
- Low-fat Yogurt
- Fermented foods (yogurt)

## DETOXIFICATION IS INHIBITED BY:

- Antidepressants
- Antihistamines
- Bacterial toxins
- Aging

## DIGESTIVE ENZYME DEFICIENCY AND INTESTINAL DYSBIOSIS

Insufficient digestion of food can lead to improperly or partially-digested food proteins entering the blood stream. These improperly digested foreign proteins can initiate an autoimmune or immune inflammatory reaction, whereby we make antibodies that attack our own body. This process, intestinal dysbiosis, can aggravate many skin conditions such as psoriasis, rosacea, acne and eczema.

In addition, frequent use of powerful antibiotics– used to treat infections and present in our food supply– combined with high fat, low fiber diets, can result in damage to the friendly normal bacteria, typically present in our large intestine or colon. In some cases the normal, useful bacteria in the gut overgrow and produce toxins which then enter the blood stream and again cause an immune, inflammatory reaction which can damage the skin.

How to restore balance to the intestinal flora? By decreasing fat in the diet, increasing fiber and yogurt and other fermented foods high in lactobacillis and the detoxification regimen listed above, as suggested by Dr. Meschino.

## WOMEN'S HORMONAL BALANCE – PRE-MENOPAUSAL

The female sex hormones, estrogen and progesterone, discussed in Chapter 3, have important effects on the skin. High estrogen – to – progesterone ratios are associated with PMS, fibrocystic breast disease, uterine fibroids, and endometriosis. Factors which can aggravate a high estrogen/progestin ratio are the following (26):

| Causes of High Estrogen/ Progestin | Improve Estrogen/ Progestin Balance |
|---|---|
| High fat diet | Low fat, high fiber diet |
| Low fiber intake | Aerobic exercise |
| Intestinal dysbiosis | Correct intestinal dysbiosis |
| Poor liver detoxification | Improve detoxification |
| Corpus luteum failure – | Black Cohash |
| (Ovarian failure) | Soy Isoflavones |
|  | Gamma-Oryzanol |

# Peri- and Post-menopausal

As discussed in Chapter 3, menopause brings a 90% decline in estrogen, and 66% decline in progesterone. These hormonal declines cause many of the symptoms of menopause. The well known symptoms are hot flashes, sweats, insomnia, anxiety and irritability.

While estrogen therapy or hormone replacement therapy (HRT) can abate the symptoms associated with menopause, there are risks associated with HRT. HRT has been shown to be associated with increase in the risk of breast cancer, heart attack, stroke and possibly ovarian cancer. Furthermore, in pre-menopausal women who have had breast cancer, estrogen suppression therapy with drugs such as Tamoxafin can also result in menopausal symptoms that have a profound aging effect on the skin of these younger women.

The following holistic or alternative therapies have been successful in Europe and Asia and do not come with the risks of HRT (27):

• Black Cohash 160 mg per day
• Soy Isoflavones 50-75 mg per day
• Gamma-Oryzanol 300 mg per day

# OTHER IMPORTANT ANTI-AGING HORMONES

Hormones are complex, highly biologically active substances that should only be used under the direction of a physician, preferably an endocrinologist. The unfortunate lesson we learned from HRT and estrogens is that hormones can stimulate the growth of cancer. Hormones should be used only when you have a documented deficiency which has been determined by testing for levels of hormones in your blood. The following discussion is for informational purposes and not a recommendation that you take these substances without a doctor's prescription.

# DEHYDROEPIANDROSTERONE (DHEA)

DHEA is the most common steroid hormone in the body and is involved in the production of many hormones including progesterone, estrogen, and testosterone. Literature suggests that, with aging, DHEA levels fall and that restoration of DHEA can result in improved immune function, restoration of lean muscle mass, and improvement in the many bodily functions that decline with aging. The problem is that if you are not deficient and you take this hormone, bad things can happen.

Have you heard of the muscular body builders who have atrophied testicles and cannot produce sperm? Abuse of DHEA is the culprit. A doctor friend of mine once told me he was taking DHEA for its anti-aging properties and he was kind enough to send me a bottle. Several months later, he told me he had developed prostate cancer. Coincidence, you say? Maybe, but the pills went into the trash. The FDA is trying hard to control the abuse of this powerful and too-readily-available hormone.

## HUMAN GROWTH HORMONE (HGH)

HGH has dramatic age reversing effects especially when given to people who are deficient in this hormone. Improvement in skin, lean body muscle mass, energy, libido, and general well-being are reported. However, as I pointed out in Chapter 3, HGH stimulates cell division and cancer is unregulated cell division. Doctor Andy Guay, a respected endocrinologist at Lahey Clinic, fears that taking HGH when you do not have a documented deficiency could turn on cells predisposed to cancer. If you might be interested in taking HGH, see an endocrinologist and have your blood levels tested. According to expert medical opinion, oral HGH preparations do not work.

For HGH to be effective, you need to take daily injections, which is a good thing because it discourages most people. Don't be ripped off by those Internet "pop ups" that promise you the fountain of youth by taking HGH pills or spray. Taking HGH pills is like putting aspirin on the top of your head for a headache!

## THYROID HORMONE

If you are deficient in thyroid hormone you are hypothyroid and must be under the care of an endocrinologist. If you are clinically deficient, thyroid hormone

will improve your bodily functions. If you are not deficient, thyroid hormone can hurt you, so don't take it!

## MELATONIN

As discussed in Chapter 3, melatonin, produced
by the pineal gland, is an important antioxidant that
specifically has protective effects on our immune system that prevents inflammation. Stress reduces our
melatonin level. Melatonin is readily available in tablet
form, and widely used as a sleep aid and to prevent "jet
lag." Studies have shown that melatonin supplementation with 0.5mg to 5mg. is safe (9). Transdermal
patches are also available.

## FOOD - YOU ARE WHAT YOU EAT

It is obvious that our diet plays a profound role
in our overall health and in the aging process. There
are excellent books on healthy eating and painstaking-
ly detailed descriptions of wholesome anti-aging diets
full of antioxidants and other important elements (18,

19). Check out those sources for detailed menu plans. The following are general dietary but critical guidelines for you to follow if you are serious about preventing – and possibly reversing – aging changes to your facial skin:

- Eat more fish, especially cold water fish such as salmon
- Eat more brightly-colored and cruciferous vegetables
- Eat more fiber
- Eat more soy products
- Eat less animal and hydrogenated fats
- Eat less refined sugar
- Drink less alcohol

I am aware that some authors today are telling you to eat, drink, and be merry. I suggest you look at the body type of the authors and if you are thin, healthy, active, and have a genetic profile compatible with longevity, then you are blessed and you may survive ignoring important dietary principles. For the rest of us mere mortals, dietary modification is an essential component for healthy longevity.

Avoid high sources of free radicals. Known sources of free radicals (28) are:

- UV light from the sun
- Cigarette smoke
- Alcohol
- Smoked or barbequed foods
- Nitrosamines (bacon and other preserved foods)
- Heavy metals – lead etc.
- X-rays
- Sugar
- Pesticides

## NUTRITIONAL ANTI-AGING CHECKLIST FOR YOUR SKIN AND FACE (A CHEAT SHEET):

### For All Skin Types
- Reduce intake of high animal fat products (meat and dairy) which lowers (AA) Arachidonic Acid.
- Reduce intake of vegetable oils which include corn, safflower seed and mixed vegetable oils which lower (LA) Linoleic Acid (High amounts of LA convert to AA).

- Do not drink alcohol.
- Reduce intake of hydrogenated fats.
- Reduce intake of refined sugars.
- Do not smoke.
- Increase intake of cruciferous vegetables which include broccoli, cauliflower and cabbage.
- Increase soy based products.
- Increase protein by having a soy – or whey – based protein shake daily.
- Drink 10 glasses of water daily.
- Increase intake of fruits high in vitamin C. Oranges are an excellent choice.
- Increase intake of vegetables. The more colorful, the better.
- Increase intake of fish. Salmon is an excellent choice and is high in Omega 3 oil.
- Wear sunscreen with an SPF of at least 15 and reapply it throughout the day if you are outdoors.

## ANTIOXIDANTS

- Vitamin C 1000 mg
- Vitamin E 400 IU.

- Beta Carotene 10,000 IU
- Selenium 100 mcg
- Zinc 15 mg
- Lycopene 6 mg
- Lutein 6 mg

## DAILY DETOX PLAN

- Cruciferous vegetables
- Oranges (contain Limonene, which is a flavinoid)
- Soy isoflavenes
- Soy Extract (supplement in a protein shake)
- Milk Thistle (a powerful detoxifier) – 150 mg up to 600 mg
- Vitamin C 1,000 mg
- Indole – 3 Carbinol – 25 up to 100 mg
- Reishi Mushroom Extract 30 mg up to 120mg
- Astragalus 100 mg up to 400 mg
- Low-fat yogurt and other fermented foods that deliver good bacteria
- Fiber

## WOMEN'S HORMONAL BALANCE

- Black Cohosh  160mg
- Soy Extract  500mg
- Gamma-oryzanol  300mg

## MEN'S PROSTATE BALANCE

- Saw Palmetto 320mg twice a day
- Pygeum Africanum 100mg twice a day
- Beta-sitosterol 65mg twice a day
- Soy extract 200mg twice a day
- Stinging Nettle 30mg twice a day
- Lycopene extract 12.5mg a day

## CHANGE YOUR LIFESTYLE

Modification of your lifestyle is one of the most important and effective steps you can take to improve your overall health and prevent aging. Avoiding alcohol, tobacco, and recreational drugs are essential for good health. Want proof? Look into the face of someone who abuses these things and you will be immediately convinced of the terrible effects of these toxins on the beauty and vitality of the human face.

## STRESS AND THE SEDENTARY LIFESTYLE — OUR MOST SELF-DESTRUCTIVE BEHAVIORS

Stress is a major factor in the production of many modern diseases, including aging. Chronic stress elevates the levels of cortisol in our body and as we learned in Chapter 3, cortisol is referred to as the age-accelerating hormone. Giampappa (19) writes that the primary source of stress in our life is "time urgency," the feeling we get when we set ourselves up to accomplish three or four tasks when we have the time to do just one.

In addition, especially for those of us who live or work in large metropolitan areas, crowding, noise, crime, and a steady diet of anxiety-provoking news makes it nearly impossible to maintain a peaceful state of mind. Many are finding that meditation and yoga are helpful antidotes for stress, a notion that is supported by some scientific medical studies (29).

## EXERCISE

Exercise is essential for good health and is one of the most effective anti-aging strategies. Some intriguing new research suggests that intensive "weekend warrior" exercise is counterproductive to good health. More moderate forms of exercise such as resistance weight training, moderate anaerobic exercise, walking, and yoga are better for our bodies and have more meaningful health and longevity promoting benefits. There are hundreds of books on exercise, but Dr. Giampappa's exercise program is specifically geared toward anti-aging and is backed by sound scientific evidence (Reference 19 Chapter 5).

The most important points about exercise are:

* Commitment – Decide that you are going to incorporate some form of exercise into each day.
* Stretch – Before and after you exercise.

- Resistance – Include some weight training in your routine. Repetitions are more important than the amount of weight.

- Aerobic exercise – Important for your heart and to release endorphins which improve your mood. Include a 30 minute period in which your heart rate increases to the safe level for your age and condition.

- Yoga – The health benefits of yoga are becoming widely recognized and many gyms now offer programs.

## SPIRITUALITY — THE KEY TO HEALTHY LONGEVITY AND A RADIANT FACE

For me, it is easier to define spirituality by stating what it is not. Many define the whole person as consisting of the body/mind/spirit. Spirituality is something we experience that is not in the realm of the body or the mind. Spirituality is a profoundly personal experience. Religion in any form is one way in which many people understand or express their personal concept of spirit, but although all people have a spiritual component to their being, not all people are religious.

The reason I include a discussion of spirituality here is because I believe, based on my 30 years of experience as a doctor, that spiritually-connected people handle most forms of stress more effectively. As we know, stress is a major factor in accelerating the aging of our skin and body. The importance of spirituality in promoting good health and recovering from illness or injury is increasingly being recognized by the contemporary medical community (30).

A recent study showed that a large number of our younger generation of college students place a high importance on spirituality. In a survey of third year college students in the United States, 58% felt that integrating spirituality in life is very important or essential. 77% of those responded that they pray; 73% said their spiritual/religious beliefs helped them develop their identities (31). In addition, millions of people worldwide have been released from the burden of addiction to drugs, food, alcohol, and other destructive behaviors by 12-step programs, which are all based on spirituality and belief in a higher power.

No one can explain why, but spirituality elevates us. I know a spiritual person when I meet one. I'm sure you do too. To me, spirituality requires humility and the acknowledgement that, no matter what our abilities are, there is a higher power, force, consciousness, or whatever you want to call it that is overwhelmingly benign. If we acknowledge it, we will be released from the burden of self-will. Failure to acknowledge a force greater than ourselves leaves us with the horrendous burden of being responsible for many things over which we really have no control. That burden, in my opinion, creates stress, anxiety and worry – all of which are not only reflected on our face by frown lines and worry lines but also negatively impact our entire body.

I'm referring to coronary artery disease, heart attacks, high blood pressure, stroke, mental illness, addictions and who knows how many more stress-related diseases. So I strongly urge you to incorporate your own spiritual program into your daily life. There are so many to choose from: organized Western reli-gions, Buddhism, you name it. For some, it may mean communing with nature or simply enjoying a beautiful painting. For me, the essential ingredient is a belief in some higher power that is responsible for our existence and experience. Armed with this humility, we can be open to experience the wonderful opportunities that are presented to us. Freed from the bonds of self-will, we will be less stressed and happier and our faces will show it. We will age less harshly and certainly in a less stressful and more healthful way.

Isn't it fascinating that we have been given the miracle of Botox® to erase frown lines and worry lines, but we cannot use this drug to reduce smile lines, because to do so would deform the face? There is a message in there for those willing to listen!

## References

1. Lim, H.W., Naylor, M., Honigsmann, H., et al. American academy of dermatology consensus conference on UVA protection of sunscreens: summary and recommendations. J. Am. Acad. Dermatol. 44: 505, 2001

2. DiGironimo, G. Skin cancer update: sunning yourself to death. Skin & Aging. 10: 16, 2002

3. Tuleya, S. Skin cancer and photo-aging update. Skin & Aging. 11:40, 2003

4. Pinnell, S. R. Cutaneous photo-damage, oxidative stress, and topical antioxidant protection. J. Am. Acad. Dermatol. 48: 1, 2003

5.  Fischer, T. and Elsner, E. The antioxidative potential of melatonin in the skin. In Thiele, J. and Elsner, P. (Eds,), Oxidants and antioxidants in cutaneous biology. Curr Probl Dermatol. Vol. 29, Basil:Karger, 2001. Pp. 165-174.

6.  Draelos, Z. D. Evaluating Vitamin Formulations. J. Aesthetic Dermatol. Cos. Surg. 1: 121, 1999.

7.  Del Rosso, J. Q. Topical retinoid therapy. Skin & Aging. 10: 50, 2002

8.  Fitzpatrick, R. E. and Rostan, E.F. Double blind, half face study comparing topical Vitamin C and vehicle for rejuvenation of photo-damage. Dermatol. Surg. 28: 231, 2002

9.  Klatz, R. and Goldman, R. Stopping the Clock Longevity for the New Millennium, 2nd Ed. North Bergen, N. J. : Basic Health Publications, 2002. Pp. 188-192

10. Ibid. Pp. 163-167

11. Ibid. Pp. 216-219

12. Ibid. Pp. 167-172

13. Ibid Pp. 198-202

14. Khatta, M., Alexander, B.S., Krichten, C.M., et al. The effect of coenzyme Q10 in patients with congestive heart failure. Ann. Intern. Med. 132: 636, 2000.

15. Watson, P.S., Scalia, G.M., Galbraith, A. et al. Lack of effect of coenzyme Q on left ventricular function in patients with congestive heart failure. J. Am. Coll. Cardiol. 33: 1549, 1999.

16. Bliznakov, E.G. Coenzyme Q10 lipid-lowering drugs (statins) and cholesterol a present day Pandora's Box. J. A. N. A. 5: 32, 2002.

17. Packer, L., Witt, E.H., Tritschler, H.J. Alpha-lipoic acid as a biological antioxidant. Free Rad. Biol. Med. 19: 227, 1995.

18. Perricone, N. The Perricone Prescription, 1st Ed. New York, 2002. Pp. 78.

19. Giampapa, V., Pero, R., and Zimmerman, M. The Anti-aging Solution, 1st Ed. Hoboken: Wiley, 2004. Pp. 138.

20. Ibid. Pp. 136.

21. Ibid. Pp. 141-144

22. Ibid. Pp. 147-148

23. Meschino, J.P. The Wrinkle Free Zone. North Bergen, NJ: Basic Health Publications, 2004.Pp. 41.

24. Ibid. Pp. 23.

25. Ibid. Pp. 58.

26. Ibid. Pp. 94.

27. Ibid. Pp. 134.

28. Ibid. Pp. 25-30.

29. Vyas, R. and Dikshit, N. Effect of meditation on respiratory system, cardio-vascular system, and lipid profile. Indian J. Physiol. Pharmacol. 46: 487, 2002.

30. Dossy, L. Prayer and medical science. Arch. Int. Med. 160: 1735, 2000.

31. College students express strong interest in spirituality and high levels of tolerance for religious diversity and the non-religious. AAC & U News. Feb. 2004.

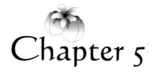

# Chapter 5

# HOW TO REVERSE FACIAL AGING — DOCTOR SECKEL'S 6-STEP PROGRAM

So far, we've focused on the factors that cause our faces to age and on the nutritional and life-style modifications that are necessary if you are seriously committed to maintaining a youthful facial appearance. In the remaining chapters, I will discuss specific medical and surgical treatments which can effectively reverse many facial aging changes that have already occurred.

All anti-aging treatments attempt to reverse facial aging by one of six basic methods. Let's take a look at these six main categories so that you will be better able to evaluate the incredible array of anti-aging solutions that are pushed at you by magazines, the Internet, talk shows, and in department stores.

Memorize these six basic methods for rejuvenating facial skin. When you see a new miracle cure on TV, ask yourself if the cure fits into any of the six categories and if so, how does it work? When you understand these methods you can readily decide if the proposed medication or other device could actually work.

## STEP 1

### Regenerate New Epithelium
### Correct Type I Aging Changes

For your face to look youthful, the coarse, dry damaged surface of your facial skin, the epithelium, must be restored. Exfoliation, the process of removing the damaged old, aged cells from the surface of the skin, is a very effective method for promoting the growth of shiny new healthy epithelial cells. As the old damaged cells are removed, the deeper layers of your skin make new epithelial cells, which grow to the surface. This is a most important first step in the facial rejuvenation process.

## STEP 2

### Remove Brown Spots and Telangiectasias Correct Type I Aging Changes

As discussed in Chapter 1, brown spots and telangiectasias are hallmarks of the aging face, and an early and important goal of any facial rejuvenation program must be to remove these aging blemishes. There are effective topical creams, which can bleach and lighten age spots or brown spots. Exfoliation is also important to remove pigment.

The new non-ablative lasers and other technologies discussed in Chapter 8 are very effective at removing both brown spots and telangiectasias and are major advances in the treatment of facial aging.

## STEP 3

### Regenerate New Dermal, Collagen and Elastin – Correct Type II Aging Changes

In Chapter 2, we learned that damage to and loss of the collagen and elastin in your skin results in the sagging and wrinkle formation which are so characteristic of the aged facial appearance. Almost all anti-aging therapies attempt to correct these Type II facial aging changes by restoring the collagen and elastin to your face. Some creams can, in fact, stimulate new collagen production, as can many of the "no down time" procedures discussed in Chapter 7. Lasers and other "high tech" anti-aging therapies also stimulate your facial skin to form new collagen and elastin. Later in the book, we'll discuss all of these therapies in detail.

## STEP 4

### Relax the Muscles of Facial Expression
### Correct Type II Aging changes

Worry lines, frown lines, crow's feet, lipstick lines, and bunny lines create a stressed and aged appearance to the face. Botox® is very useful for correcting these lines. Some newer topical creams may also be useful. We'll get back to this later in the book.

# STEP 5

## Fill or Camouflage Deep Facial Lines
## Correct Type II Aging Changes

The nasal-labial fold and marionette lines are very distressing facial aging changes. Face-lifting and laser resurfacing can be very effective in improving – but not totally correcting – these changes. Among the non-surgical methods, fillers can be injected under the skin to plump it up and camouflage the line.

# STEP 6

## Tighten Facial Skin
## Correct Type II Aging Changes

Although we have many therapies that have been proven to stimulate skin to form new collagen and elastin, this benefit often does not translate into a tightening effect on your skin. While laser resurfacing and face-lifting can dramatically tighten facial skin most people do not want to undergo these invasive procedures.

Recently, new technologies using radiofrequency waves and infrared light have shown promise as noninvasive methods for actually tightening the facial skin (see Chapter 8 – High Tech Facial Rejuvenation). Of course the "gold standard" for tightening the facial skin remains the face-lift and laser resurfacing.

The important point to remember is that no one type of therapy corrects all facial aging changes. That's why it is so important for you to understand how each of these therapies works. Remember, if it sounds too good to be true, it is. Effective facial rejuvenation requires a careful, step-by-step, systematic approach. Your doctor needs to be aware of all six facial rejuvenation methods and to understand how to apply them to your unique face. No one type of therapy is effective for all people.

Avoid doctors who fit the description "when your only tool is a hammer, the whole world looks like a nail." Some doctors only do one thing well and they will attempt to solve all of your aging problems with one technique, such as collagen injections, Botox®, or laser, because they don't have the skills or equipment necessary to do non-ablative therapy or surgery.

Your doctor should be knowledgeable about the whole spectrum of facial aging changes and he or she should be able to offer specific solutions for each of the aging issues that concern you, or be willing and able to refer you to someone who can.

Below is a table summarizing the logical scientifically based, medically accepted methods for reversing facial aging. I have organized these steps into a 6-step program which enables you to address each specific aging change in a logical step-wise fashion. Using this protocol you can decide which facial aging changes are present in your face and thus be able to select the appropriate therapy for your face. Armed with this knowledge you will be an informed consumer and able to decide if the therapy being offered to you by a physician really addresses your problem. This table will help you make sense out of the confusing array of modern anti-aging therapies (Table 5-1).

| ANTI-AGING TREATMENT | AGING CHANGE TREATED | TREATMENTS AVAILABLE |
|---|---|---|
| **Step 1** Exfoliation | Aged dry skin | Microdermabrasion Micro Peel® MicroLasePeel® Topical creams |
| **Step 2** Remove brown spots and telangiectasias | Blemish removal | Lasers, IPL, topical creams, exfoliation |
| **Step 3** Regenerate dermal, collagen and elastin | Plump and firm skin | Lasers, IPL, topical creams MicroLaserPeel® |
| **Step 4** Relax muscles of facial expression | Correct worry lines frown lines, crow's feet, bunny lines | Botox® ? some topical creams |
| **Step 5** Camouflage deep facial lines | Camouflage nasal-labial fold lines, marionette lines | Fillers |
| **Step 6** Tighten facial skin | Correct lose skin and wrinkles | Laser resurfacing, Face-lift surgery, Collagen remodeling (Titan®, Thermage®) |

**TABLE 5-1.**
*Doctor Seckel's 6 Step Program*

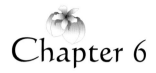

# Chapter 6

# MAGICAL POTIONS
# THE FOUNTAIN OF YOUTH

## TOPICAL SKIN CREAMS
## "THE WRINKLE CURE"®

Billions of dollars, over twenty billion a year, are spent on skin creams to prevent or reverse facial aging. Most of that money is wasted. The majority of the non pre-scription anti-aging creams do not work.

The most important thing I want you to remem-ber as you read this chapter is that there are <u>only two treatments that have been approved by the FDA as effective for reversing facial aging changes – Retin A® and laser resurfacing</u>, the latter, of course is a surgical procedure.

The competitive marketing of anti-aging skin creams has created a confounding array of products. As Dr. Klingman, the pioneer who developed Retin A®, put it, "We have a marketplace that is absolutely crazy and the consumer is left to do her own personal clinical trial to see what works" (1). The FDA requires labeling on prescription creams other than Retin A® to state in bold print: **These products do not remove or prevent wrinkles, repair sun damaged skin, reverse aging due to sun or restore your more youthful skin.** Certainly, FDA approval often lags behind the development of promising new therapies, but the FDA waits for scientifically valid clinical studies before it grants approval.

So what can you do? Consult a reputable doctor who specializes in facial aging, a dermatologist or a plastic surgeon who is informed and up-to-date on this subject. Don't rely on what you read in beauty magazines, what you hear on talk shows, or from the charming salesperson at the cosmetic counter. Set the pop up ad controls on your computer so you won't be bombarded with that annoying array of false promises that are designed to pull you in and take your money!

The worst offenders are the infomercials. Think about that word "infomercial." It is used to sucker you in. These are commercials designed to sell you a product. They add the prefix "info" instead of "com" to make you think they are providing you with valid information. Listen to what they're saying. Do they provide you with a reference reporting a clinical trial published in a medical journal? Of course not, because there is none!

I saw an infomercial on TV in which a beautiful movie star was touting the advantages of a miracle cream which was purported to be "better than Botox®." Do you realize that such spokespersons are paid for their statements and most often have never used the product? In my opinion, nowhere is this misleading type of advertising more pervasive than in the field of anti-aging creams and solutions. Why? Because this field is so hot. These entrepreneurs have read the data on the huge population of aging baby boomers who do not want to grow old, and we are ripe for the picking.

Please read this chapter carefully, and only use products for which there is some scientifically proven data to support their use. In the discussion below, I will differentiate between agents that have clinical studies to back up their claims and those that may make intuitive sense, but do not yet have the science to justify their claims. The most effective, proven skin creams and solutions require a doctor's prescription. Does this surprise you? I doubt it.

## HOW DO TOPICAL CREAMS, GELS, OINTMENTS AND SOLUTIONS CORRECT AGING CHANGES?

Topical agents can reverse facial aging changes by:
- Exfoliating or removing dead epithelial cells from the skin  surface
- Promoting the growth of new epithelial cells
- Halting the production of pigment, which causes brown spots

- Stimulating the production of new collagen in the dermis
- Blocking the production of enzymes that breakdown or destroy collagen
- Delivering antioxidants or free radical scavengers to the skin

Remember these effects occur at a submicroscopic cellular level. Don't expect visible, drastic or immediate results. The changes, produced by skin creams are subtle and are noticed only after six months or a year of continued daily use. Claims of a "face-lift in a jar" or a cream that causes "immediate plumping of the skin or lips" are nonsense, unless, of course, you have an allergic reaction to the cream.

## RETIN A®

This chemical, also known as tretinoin, is a by-product of Vitamin A synthesis and is a member of a key family of skin care medications called the retinoids. Retinoids regulate the growth of the epidermis, inhibit the formation of cancer, decrease inflammation and improve immune function. Retin A® is a prescription drug. You cannot buy it at the beauty counter. Retin A®, a drug in cream form, has been clinically proven to improve the epithelium, stimulate new collagen production, prevent collagen breakdown and lessen pigmentation (2). Why would you want to use anything else?

Retin A® can be mixed with Hydroquinone 4%, a bleaching cream to enhance the removal of pigment or brown spots which improves the anti-aging effectiveness of Retin A®. In addition, when used in conjunction with microdermabrasion (we'll discuss this more in the next chapter) Retin A®'s penetration and effectiveness are enhanced.

Retin A® is too irritating for many people, however. Also, you must wear sun block while using Retin A® because the drug can sensitize your skin to the sun. Thus, sun block and skin protection (such as a hat and large sunglasses) are essential. Newer, less-irritating compounds are Renova® and Retin A Micro®. Retin A® comes in different strengths – 0.01%, 0.025%, 0.05%, and 0.1%. I typically start patients on 0.025% to see if they can tolerate the product well, and if they can, I gradually increase the strength. Tazorac® and Avage®, two other products containing tazarotine, a retinoid which has been very effective for treating psoriasis and acne, are now approved for their anti-aging effects.

# RETINOLS

Retinols are available as over-the-counter products, no prescription necessary. Although their effectiveness is a matter of controversy among dermatologists, these compounds, once applied, are converted in your skin to retinoesters and small quantities of tretinoin or Retin A®. Combining Retinol 0.3% with Hydroquinone 4% (Epiquin®) is effective in resolving fine lines, pigment and improving skin texture (3). Retinols are not as strong as Retin A® and, therefore, can be used by many people who cannot tolerate the stronger products.

# ALPHA HYDROXY ACIDS (AHAS)

The AHAs – glycolic acid and lactic acid – are derived from fruit and milk sugars. The AHA most commonly used is glycolic acid, which is widely added to over-the-counter skin creams and by estheticians and doctors to perform skin peels to reverse skin aging damage and pigmentation.

AHAs produce exfoliation and stimulate the production of new collagen in the dermis, so they are a valuable component of most anti-aging skin care regimens. A recent study also showed that glycolic acid treatment of the skin increased the hyaluronic acid (HA) content of both the epidermis and dermis, a very exciting finding since, as we know, the loss of HA is an important cause of dryness in aged skin (4).

Don't let their benign origins fool you, though! AHAs can be very irritating. The FDA estimates there are 10,000 adverse reactions to AHA- containing products each year, reactions that can include redness, swelling of the eyes, rash, itching and skin discoloration (5). The stronger solutions of AHAs are used by doctors to produce a chemical peel, which blisters or removes the epithelium and irritates the dermis in order to encourage more new collagen production.

Skin care products sold over-the-counter, which contain glycolic or lactic acid, contain, at most, only 10% AHAs. Trained cosmetologists may use products which contain 20-30% AHAs. Doctors may use products with as much as 50-70% AHAs, but at these concentrations, a deep chemical peel is produced.

I frequently use AHAs, both in prescription and non-prescription forms for patients who cannot tolerate Retin A®. The Cosmetic Ingredient Review Panel (5) concludes that AHA's, glycolic and lactic acid are safe for you the consumer when:

- The AHA concentration is 10% or less
- The pH is 3.5 or higher
- The product contains sunscreen or the label clearly recommends that you use sunscreen.

## VITAMIN C - L ASCORBIC ACID

Vitamin C is an important antioxidant which, in the form of L ascorbic acid, can be applied topically to the skin. When Vitamin C ester is put in a lipophilic (fat loving) solution it may be possible to deliver it directly to the skin (6). As you remember, the skin cells have fat in their cell walls, and the Vitamin C ester must be in a solution which can penetrate this fatty barrier to get into the skin to have an effect.

Vitamin C ester has multiple anti-aging effects. It's a free radical scavenger, it promotes new collagen formation, and it actively protects skin from the aging effects of UV radiation in sunlight, above and beyond the benefit provided by sun block. This effect is enhanced by the addition of Vitamin E (7). I frequently use Vitamin C preparations on patients who cannot tolerate Retin A®, and in patients with rosacea or other inflammatory skin conditions for whom Retin A® is too irritating.

## VITAMIN E (TOCOPHEROLS AND TOCOTRIENOLS)

You'll recall from Chapters 3 and 4 that Vitamin E is one of the most powerful antioxidants and has been shown to be beneficial in combating both heart disease and cancer. Vitamin E also plays a role in protecting the skin from aging damage caused by the sun (8) when used in combination with Vitamin C in sun block. Traditionally, Vitamin E has been taken orally along with other antioxidants, but recently topical solutions containing Vitamin E have become available. Many new prescription anti-aging creams have Vitamin E and other antioxidant vitamins in their formulas.

## ALPHA LIPOIC ACID (ALA)

Recently, there has been much interest in the antioxidant ALA as a supplement useful for preventing facial aging (9). Most of the oft-quoted studies have in fact been done on rats, so definitive evidence of the usefulness of ALA in humans awaits further research. One clinical study in humans has been published which suggests that topical application of ALA can reverse textural changes in the facial skin associated with aging (10). Whether these changes are the result of epithelial cell regeneration and new collagen formation, or from some other direct effect on the skin (such as improving moisture content or swelling) need to be determined by microscopic studies of skin biopsies.

## COENZYME Q10 (UBIQUINONE, IDEBENONE)

As discussed in Chapter 4, Coenzyme Q10 is important in cellular metabolism and acts as an antioxidant to protect cell membranes from damage by free radicals. As we've learned, clinical studies on the effectiveness of Coenzyme Q10 in humans are equivocal. Although Coenzyme Q10 is being sold as a component of some topical solutions, I can find no scientifically controlled clinical studies in which it has been shown to be useful as a topical agent.

Recently there has been a great deal of publicity about a synthetic analogue of Coenzyme Q10 called Idebenone. In laboratory experiments Idebenone has proven to be a more powerful antioxidant than Coenzyme Q10. One early, yet unpublished, clinical trial on 28 patients, provided by the company that makes Prevage® a cream containing Idebenone, reports encouraging results.

# PPC (POLYENYLPHOSPHATIDYL CHOLINE)

PPC, a phospholipid (fat) with antioxidant properties, has been touted as an effective emollient and anti-aging cream (9). To my knowledge, the main therapeutic use of this agent which is documented in the scientific literature is in alcoholic liver disease in rats (11).

Thus, if you are a non-rat I would wait on controlled clinical studies in humans before I pinned my anti-aging hopes on this topical preparation! PPC, a fat containing phospholipid, may well be a good moisturizer but there are many others available, some of which are more appealing to me on a scientific basis (see Hyaluronic Acid (HA) below.)

# DMAE (DIMETHYLAMINOETHANOL) — "FACE-LIFT IN A JAR"?

Remember what I wrote about things that are too good to be true? DMAE has been recommended as a treatment for Alzheimer's disease, Tardive Dyskinesia, a movement disorder related to Parkinson's disease, and Attention Deficit Disorder. Controlled clinical studies have failed to show a demonstrable benefit of this agent in any of these conditions. Why would you expect this agent to give you a face-lift?

DMEA is a precursor of choline, which is a component of acetylcholine, the chemical released from nerves to make the facial muscles contract or tighten. The theory is, if you apply DMAE, choline synthesis will be increased, leading to increased production of acetylcholine which will result in contraction or tightening of your facial muscles, and tightening of your skin.

One recent report (12) suggested that topical DMEA did in fact tighten one side of the face in a split-face study where one side of the face was treated with DMAE and the other side was not treated.

The proposed mechanism of this tightening is contraction of the facial muscles. Do you remember from Chapter 2 what causes frown lines, worry lines and crows feet? The answer is, of course, muscle contraction! We block the action of acetylcholine with Botox® to weaken muscle contraction to get rid of your facial lines. Furthermore, what causes the skin to sag is loss of elasticity, not loss of muscle contraction.

It seems to me that the "face-lift in a jar" and Botox® work against each other. Perhaps you can use them both together. When taken orally, DMAE can have serious side effects including worsening of depression and schizophrenia. Personally, I think I would go for the face-lift!

Perhaps this compound will be used in the future to firm the skin by some not-yet- clearly understood mechanism but, at present, I am skeptical. I can assure you that DMAE is not a face-lift in a jar, which is a pre-posterous claim.

## Acetyl Hexapeptide-3 – "Better Than Botox®"?

The shameless hyperbole of the vendors of anti-aging creams casts a sorrowful shadow on what might be a promising new drug. According to the companies that sell products containing Acetyl Hexapeptide-3, it is a highly-sophisticated, genetically-engineered protein designed to block the release of acetylcholine from nerve endings. This is a mechanism for muscle relaxation similar to that of Botox®, but it occurs at a much smaller site on the cell membrane of the nerve terminal.

Manufacturers of products containing Acetyl Hexapeptide-3 claim that this chemical can be delivered through the skin in the form of a topical cream, and slowly and minimally relax the facial muscles and reduce wrinkles. Some claim that this chemical prolongs the effects of Botox®.

Unfortunately, the only article offering a clinical study showing significant results was on a website which offered to sell you their product, but failed to reference a publication for their study (info@cremedevoie.com!) Several creams, among them Avotox®, StriVectin-SD®, SerumXL®, and Creme de Vie®, claim that they contain Acetyl-Hexapeptide-3, and that these creams remove wrinkles by the above mechanism.

Again, an extensive search of the credible scientific literature failed to substantiate these claims. Perhaps this newly-manufactured protein is so new that studies have not been published, but if that is the case, I question whether or not they should be selling it to you, the consumer. Perhaps controlled clinical trials will be done to prove or disprove the effectiveness of these new creams.

The concept is very exciting, and if the claims are substantiated by controlled clinical studies, this truly will be a revolutionary new product.

## PALMITOYL PENTAPEPTIDE

Palmitoyl pentapeptide (also known as palmitoyl oligopeptide) is a new skin rejuvenation compound. Proponents claim that palmitoyl pentapeptide is at least as effective against wrinkles as retinol but it does not cause skin irritation, a common side-effect of retinoids.

Chemically speaking, palmitoyl pentapeptide is a relatively small molecule (five amino acids linked together and attached to a fatty acid) structurally related to the precursor of collagen type I (procollagen type I). Researchers found that, when added to the culture of fibroblasts (the key collagen producing skin cells), palmitoyl pentapeptide stimulated the synthesis of the key constituents of the skin matrix: collagen, elastin and glucosamnoglycans.

So far, clinical data are encouraging. One study demonstrated that palmitoyl pentapeptide was as effective as Retinol in repairing sun-damaged skin but without the side effects. So, Palmitoyl pentapeptide, with its good safety profile, may be worth a try. Palmitoyl pentapeptide may also be considered as a non-irritating fall-back option for people who develop skin irritation in response to retinoids or alpha-hydroxy acids.

## HYALURONIC ACID (HA)

As mentioned in Chapter 2, HA is a crucial moisturizing and nutrition-providing substance found throughout the skin. By age 50, we have lost much of this valuable skin component. Hyaluronic Acid (HA) has recently been in the news as filler to inject into the skin to correct wrinkles. (See the next chapter.) What I am discussing here is the use of HA in skin creams. Widely used as a humectant or moisturizer in skin creams, HA is an excellent moisturizer.

Whether or not topically applied HA is actually taken up by the dermis and contributes to the total skin content of HA is unknown. In my opinion, it is unlikely, in view of the fact that the very pure forms of HA that we inject into the skin as fillers are biodegraded in a matter of 6 to 9 months and injections have to be repeated to maintain the correction of wrinkles and deep facial lines. If we could restore the HA content of our skin, improvement in moisture content, firmness and suppleness would result.

I think it is unlikely that any cream, gel, or other topical agent can restore the HA lost by aging. Estrogen has been reported to increase HA synthesis in the skin, but the dangers of estrogen replacement out-weigh this potential benefit. Creams containing HA are wonderful moisturizers but do not pay a premium expecting the cream to reverse aging by regenerating the HA content of your skin.

## BLEACHING AGENTS

Hydroquinone 4% and Kojic acid are two very useful skin bleaching agents. Superficial pigmentation, Type I aging skin changes can be lightened by using these bleaching creams, especially when they are used in combination with a retinoid such as Retin A® or Retinol. Pigment removal is also enhanced when these agents are used in conjunction with exfoliation such as microdermabrasion (see Chapter 7.)

Hydroquinone should be stopped after six months of use as there is risk of hyperpigmentation with prolonged use. After a rest period of three to six months, hydroquinone may be used again. Three months on and three months off is another acceptable way to use Hydroquinone.

## SUMMARY

In summary, I urge you to go back and read the first few paragraphs of this chapter. The cosmetic and pharmaceutical industries have become incredibly sophisticated in their marketing approaches. They know our generation is informed and well-educated and demands to understand the science behind the claims they make about their products.

Seriously reviewing this topic was an incredible eye-opener for me. When you carefully review the claims made for many of the anti-aging products, it becomes readily apparent that there is very little hard data and few scientifically controlled clinical studies to support the incredible claims that are made about most if not all of these new "miracle" products.

What's happening is this: An exciting new theory or very early discovery is produced, packaged and marketed to you as if the anti-aging benefits are proven facts. They are not. You need to be an informed consumer, and, more than ever, you need the advice of a knowledgeable doctor to help you sort through the confusing array of claims and counter-claims. I have tried to give you a good review of this topic as I understand it, and I will summarize my findings below (Table 6-1).

| PRODUCT | ACTION | EFFECT | PROVEN TO WORK | BRAND NAMES | DR. SECKEL RECOMMENDS |
|---|---|---|---|---|---|
| Retin A® | promotes growth of new epithelium promotes new collagen | helps fine lines helps remove pigment improves the look of the skin | yes | Retin A® | yes |
| Tazarotine | same as RetinA® | same as RetinA® | yes | Tazorac® Avage® | yes |
| Retinols | same as Retin A | same as Retin A | when used with Hydroxyquinone | Epiquin® | yes |
| Hydroxyquinone | removes pigment | lightens brown spots | yes | Claripel®, Epiquin®, Glyquin® | yes |
| AHA's, Glycolic Acid | exfoliation, collagen production | improves fine lines | yes | Glyquin® | yes |
| Vitamin C ester (L Ascorbic Acid) | antioxidant free radical scavenger, promotes collagen production, protection from sun | improves fine lines improves skin texture | yes | Vitamin C Serum® | yes |

**TABLE 6-1.**

| PRODUCT | ACTION | EFFECT | PROVEN TO WORK | BRAND NAMES | DR. SECKEL RECOMMENDS |
|---|---|---|---|---|---|
| Vitamin E | antioxidant and sun protectant especially in combination with Vitamin C | prevents aging changes caused by sun | yes | Glyquin® | yes |
| ALA Alpha Lipoic Acid | antioxidant | improves skin texture | no | ? | no |
| Coenzyme Q10 Ubiquinone | antioxidant | unknown | no | ? | no |
| Idebenone | antioxidant | unknown | no | Prevage® | no |
| PPC (polyenyl phosphatidylcholine) | antioxidant moisturizer | improved skin texture | no | | no |
| DMAE (Dimethylaminoethaol) | stimulates facial muscle contraction | "face-lift in a jar" | no | | no |
| Acetyl Hexapeptide-3 | relaxes facial muscles | "Better Than Botox®" | no | Avotox®, StriVectin-SD®, Serum XL®, & Creme de Vie® | no |

TABLE 6-1. CONTINUED

| PRODUCT | ACTION | EFFECT | PROVEN TO WORK | BRAND NAMES | DR. SECKEL RECOM- MENDS |
|---|---|---|---|---|---|
| Palmitoyl Pentapep tide | stimulates collagen and elastin production | "Gentle" Retinol effects | no | ? | no |
| Hyaluro- nic Acid (HA) | moisturiz- ing skin compo- nent | moistur- izer, softens skin | no anti- aging effect or replace- ment of skin HA proven | | yes |

**TABLE 6-1. CONTINUED**

Personally, all of my patients are on a topical cream or solution containing at least one of the following components which have been scientifically proven to work:

• Retin A®
• Alpha Hydroxy Acids (AHA)-Glycolic Acid
• Vitamin C ester (L Ascorbic Acid)
• Vitamin E

Topical creams and solutions are only one very small skirmish in the facial anti-aging battle, however. Their appeal is that they are so easy to use, but you know all to well at this stage of your life that nothing really good comes easily! Read on.

# REFERENCES

1. Murphy, R. Cosmaceuticals: can they support the claims? Skin & Aging. 9: 1, 2001.

2. Nyirady, J., Bergfeld, W., Ellis, C., et al. Tretinoin cream o.o2% for the treatment of photo-damaged facial skin: a review of 2 double-blind clinical studies. Cutis. 68: 135, 2001.

3. Draelos, D. Evaluating vitamin formulations. J. Aesth. Dermatol. and Cos. Surg. 1: 121, 1999.

4. Bernstein, E. F., Lee, J., Brown, D. B., et al. Glycolic acid treatment increases type 1 collagen mRNA and hyaluronic acid content of human skin. Dermatol. Surg. 27: 5, 2001.

5. Kurtzwell, P. Alpha hydroxyl acids for skincare-smooth sailing or rough seas. FDA Consumer Magazine. March-April: 298, 1999.

6. Perricone, N. The Perricone Prescription, 1st Ed. New York, 2002. Pp. 113.

7. Greul, A. K., Grundmann,J. U., Heinrich, F. et al. Photoprotection of UV-irradiated human skin: an antioxidative combination of vitamins E and C, carotenoids, selenium and proanthocyanidins. Skin Pharmacol. Appl. Skin Physiol. 15: 307, 2002.

8. Lupo, M. P., Antioxidants and vitamins in cosmetics. Clin. in Dermatol.19: 467, 2001.

9.  Perricone, N., The wrinkle cure. 1st Ed. New York: Warner, 2001. Pp. 67-80

10. Beitner, H. Randomized, placebo controlled, double blind study on the efficacy of a cream containing 5% alpha-lipoic acid related to photo-aging of facial skin. Br. J. Dermatol. 149: 841, 2003.

11. Navder, K. P., and Baraona, E., Polyenylphosphatidylcholine attenuates alcohol-induced fatty liver and hyperlipemia in rats. J. of Nutr. 127:1800, 1997.

12. Uhoda, I., Faska, N., Robert, C., Split face study on the cutaneous tensile effect of 2- dimethylaminoethanol (deanol) gel. Skin Res. Technol. 8: 164, 2002.

13. Casey, D.E. Mood alterations during deanol therapy. Psychopharmacology (Berl). 62: 187, 1979.

# Chapter 7

# No Down Time Facial Anti-aging Procedures

The treatments covered in this chapter are my *absolute favorite* non-surgical therapies for facial rejuvenation. They are perfect for the busy lifestyle we all have which does not permit us to have "down time" away from family, work, or friends. More importantly, they work! You either see an immediate result, or at most, you'll see results in a couple of weeks (Botox®). If it is not an immediately visible result, you will feel the difference in your skin very soon after the procedure.

For a person with a surgical temperament like me (and most of my patients), waiting for months, looking hopefully in the mirror to see minor skin improvements (if we're lucky) from creams and lotions, is not an option!

Within this group of therapies are some of the most beneficial, effective, modern treatments in existence today, provided they are performed by someone who is expert in their use. By expert I mean a doctor or a medical professional (nurse, physician assistant (PA), or medical aesthetician) who is under the doctor's supervision. A supervising doctor should be present in the facility while the treatment is being done. The idea that a doctor can supervise from a distant location is ludicrous and is simply a ploy used by entrepreneurs to make more money at the expense of the quality and safety of your care. If you go to a facility and the doctor is not on the premises, leave. Quickly.

The whole idea of doctor supervision is to make certain you are receiving the proper therapy and to guarantee your safety if something goes wrong. Treatments that involve injection such as Botox® and fillers must be done by a physician. If you doubt me skip ahead and read Chapter 9 – "Don't Let Just Anyone Touch Your Face."

## Microdermabrasion — Dermagenesis®

Microdermabrasion is my favorite "no down time" procedure. A medical aesthetician in my office passes a small tube across your face. The tube has small sand-like particles rushing through it. A small opening in the tube is placed on your skin. The skin is gently sucked into the tube, into the stream of particles. These rushing particles resurface or exfoliate your skin, removing sebum, unblocking pores and removing dead skin cells and superficial pigment.

The microdermabrasion procedure is performed by a medical aesthetician in my office under my supervision (Figure 7-1). We use the microdermabrasion machine made by Dermagenisis® which is capable of a deep effective peel. The benefits of having this procedure done in a physician's office are:

- A doctor is present and can write a prescription for a topical that works
- Stronger peel solutions can be used if necessary

- Some of you need a MicroPeel® or other treatment not available in a salon. In a physicians office the appropriate treatment can be determined and offered to you
- In the rare instance in which something goes wrong the doctor is available immediately
- Certain medical conditions and/or medications require special attention and modification of the procedure

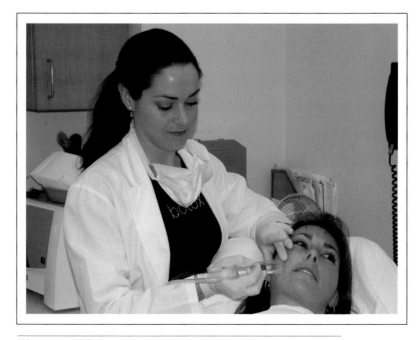

**FIGURE 7-1.**

*Microdermabrasion is a painless "no down time" procedure with wonderful results for your skin.*

- Prophylactic prescription anti-Herpes medication is required for those individuals prone to Herpes outbreaks on the face
- Often pre-cancerous or cancerous lesions on the face can be detected early by a physician

Following microdermabrasion, your skin looks and feels smooth and refreshed. Because dead skin has been removed, topical treatments like Retin A®, Retinol, AHAs, and Vitamin C can more easily penetrate the skin. Skin biopsies have shown that, following six microdermabrasion treatments, the epithelium is thicker and healthier-looking and there is an increase in superficial dermal collagen. Both are important goals in any anti-aging treatment (1). In addition to providing significant microscopic improvement in the skin, microdermabrasion patients report high satisfaction with the treatment in clinical studies (2, 3). This treatment effectively removes superficial hyperpigmentation when used in conjunction with the appropriate prescription topical agents. The results after a series of treatments over several months are truly remarkable and gratifying (Figure 7-2).

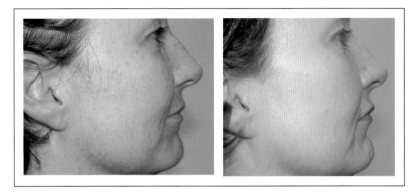

**FIGURE 7-2.**

*A patient with hyperpigmentation and Type I aging changes before (left) and after (right) a series of microdermabrasion treatments.*

Microdermabrasion is most effective if used in an overall, multi-step rejuvenation program involving prescription topical creams and other more invasive procedures, which only can be done in a physician's office.

## MICROPEEL®

MicroPeel® refers to a combination of derma-planing (scraping dead skin off your face) and applying a dilute AHA (glycolic acid) following the derma-planing. This is referred to as "the lunchtime peel" because pinkness is minimal and you can go back to work after this is done. This procedure was developed by Biomedic® as a useful adjunct to anti-aging therapies and is useful in patients who have sensitive skin who cannot tolerate the microdermabrasion.

This procedure is only available in a physician's office, as Biomedic® does not allow their product to be

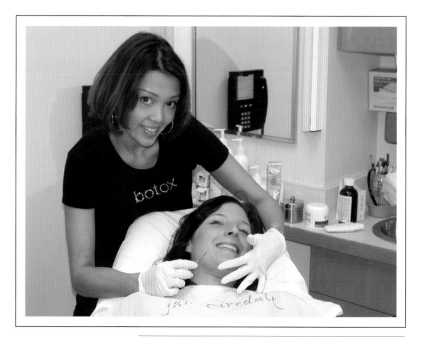

**FIGURE 7-3.**

*Medical aesthetician performs a MicroPeel®
in doctor's office*

sold to salons and spas (Figure 7-3). This is a safety issue and Biomedic® is to be congratulated for putting patient safety and ethics ahead of profit.

The benefit to you, the patient, is that in a physician's office, you will receive the appropriate procedure and if needed, a prescription for a topical which will enhance the benefit of the MicroPeel® procedure.

It is also very helpful for acne patients. Micro Peel Plus® is also available with added salicylic acid, which makes the peel go a little bit deeper for more effective exfoliation and the stimulation of new collagen growth in the dermis.

## Superficial Chemical Peels

Superficial peels with AHAs of 20-30% or salicylic acid can be applied by medical aestheticians in a doctor's office under the supervision of a physician. These peels provide exfoliation, removal of superficial pigment, and can also stimulate new collagen production.

The deeper peels, with high percentage AHAs (50-70%), TCA peels and phenol peels are considered surgical procedures, to be performed by a physician. These are not minimally invasive. Deeper peels, such as these, can be very effective, but there is significant down time.

I do not use deep peels because the risk of scarring and hypo-pigmentation (whitening of the treated skin) are too great. Most physicians today prefer laser resurfacing if a deeper peel is needed. This is a much more controllable, less risky form of facial resurfacing (see Chapter 8). Some doctors get beautiful results with the deeper peels and are more experienced than I am in their use. I have simply seen too many patients who suffered complications after another doctor has done their peel, and at that point, unfortunately, there is nothing I can do to help them.

## MicroLaserPeel®

MicroLaserPeel® is a new, superficial form of Erbium laser peel, which is very exciting. Whereas microdermabrasion can remove 5-8 microns of skin (a micron is one thousandth of a millimeter or one millionth of a meter), an Erbium MicroLaserPeel® can remove 10 to 20 microns of skin without producing significant down time. The goal is exfoliation and irritation of the dermis to produce new collagen, and to enhance the penetration of the topical agents such as Retin A®, Retinols, AHAs, or Vitamin C. Deeper, 30 to 40 micron MicroLaserPeels® are more effective, but will leave you pink for three to five days.

The Erbium MicroLaserPeel® is a procedure that is more effective than microdermabrasion because the treatment can remove more tissue and effect the dermal collagen more intensely to stimulate new collagen production. Deeper pigmentation can be removed by this technique than by microdermabrasion alone. While the skin may be pink for a few days depending on the depth of treatment the recovery is not nearly as prolonged as it is with laser resurfacing (see Chapter 9). Results are very gratifying (Figure 7-4). The duration of pinkness depends on the depth of the peel:

- 10 micron peel _____ pink for 1-2days
- 20 micron peel _____ pink for 2-3 days
- 40 micron peel _____ pink for 5-7 days

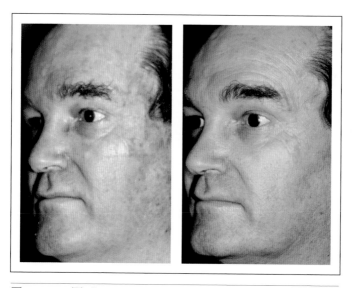

**FIGURE 7-4.**

*Before (left) and after (right) a 40 micron MicroLaserPeel®. The patient's face was pink for one week. (Photo courtesy of Bruce M. Friedman, M.D. and Sciton®)*

# BOTOX®

Botox® is the most revolutionary and effective facial anti-aging treatment since the advent of laser resurfacing. Unlike laser resurfacing, there is no down time with the procedure, which, along with the effectiveness of Botox® accounts for its incredible popularity. Yes, the name Botox® is short for botulinum toxin, a toxin produced by the bacteria Clostridium Botulinum. It was discovered in 1895 and purified as botulinum toxin A (the type we use today) in 1946. It was first used in the late 1970's to treat torticollis and other severe forms of muscle spasm and was found to be very safe and effective.

In the 1980's, doctors Jean and Alastair Carruthers noticed that when they used Botox® to treat patients with ocular spasm (spasm of the eyelid) the wrinkles or crow's feet around the treated eye disappeared (4). These results encouraged doctors to use Botox® to treat the lines of facial expression, frown lines, worry lines, and crow's feet. The cosmetic use of Botox® was approved by the FDA in April 2002.

Botox® works by weakening the muscles of facial expression. When you contract or tighten one of the muscles of facial expression, the nerve which connects with the muscle releases a chemical called acetylcholine. The acetylcholine then stimulates the muscle to contract or tighten. Botox® works by blocking the effect of acetylcholine on the muscle, and causes the muscle to relax and quit pulling on the skin. When the muscle stops pulling on the skin, the wrinkle caused by the muscle pull goes away. Importantly, the muscles of facial expression function to produce an expression on your face.

The muscles of facial expression that we treat with Botox® are not involved in chewing or other important functional tasks. If they were, we would not use Botox® on them. Botox® also works well on the bunny lines, those little lines at the base of your nose when you squint or wrinkle your nose. The part of your eyelid muscle that is important for eye closure is not treated with Botox®; we treat only the outer part of that muscle which causes the crow's feet because the part directly beneath the eyelid is crucial for eye lid closure and we do not want to interfere with this extremely important function. (Figure 7-5).

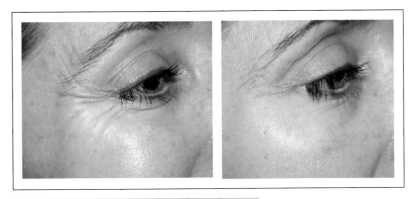

**FIGURE 7-5.**

*Before (left) and 3 weeks (right) after Botox® injection for "crows feet" (patient is actively smiling in both photographs.)*

Botox® injections are quick and relatively pain-less, especially when the area to be injected is iced first and a small 32 gauge needle is used.

Doctors who are expert at the use of Botox® can also use Botox® to lessen lipstick lines and some of the deep furrows below the lip on the chin. Only small amounts, two or three IU's (International Units) are used in these areas.

Correction of the lines of facial expression is not permanent, so Botox® injections must be repeated. The initial injection lasts three to six months, but the second injection often lasts six to nine months. The effect of Botox® on the muscle seems to be cumulative in my experience, raising the possibility that after two to three years of use, the muscles will have atrophied and will be weak enough that repeat injections may not be necessary. At the present time, however, you should assume that you will continue to need Botox® injections every 6 to 9 months for as long as you want the lines to be gone.

It is essential that the physician who injects Botox® be experienced in the injection techniques for this drug. Botox® must be accurately placed within the muscle for it to work. The muscular anatomy of the face is very complex and injections can easily be placed too deep (below the muscle), or too superficially (in the dermis.) In either case, the injection will not work as well and you will be unhappy with the result. This is not something that a nurse or anyone other than a physician should be doing. It looks so simple, but technique is very important.

If Botox® is placed into the wrong muscle, your eyelid can droop or your smile can become crooked. Ask the right questions when you seek this treatment. Adverse reactions that have been reported are headaches (13%), nausea (3%), and flu-like syndrome (2%), but whether they are related to the Botox® is unknown. Three percent of patients in initial studies had temporary eyelid droop lasting three to six weeks, but in my opinion, eyelid droop can be avoided by proper injection technique.

Botox® injections sting, but the discomfort can be significantly reduced by icing the area prior to injection and diluting the Botox® with a preservative containing saline. Botox® is expensive. Botox® comes from the manufacturer as a powder which must be refrigerated. It must be mixed and diluted with saline (salt water) prior to injection and after it is diluted, it must be kept refrigerated. The company that makes Botox® recommends that the diluted, refrigerated Botox® be used within two weeks, or it loses much of its effectiveness.

Treatments are charged by the unit of Botox®, usually around $20 per unit. A typical initial treatment uses 25 units, which costs $500. Fifty units is usually the maximum treatment recommended for one session. In my practice, 50 units could easily treat frown lines, worry lines, crow's feet and bunny lines. Very small amounts (1-3 units) are used around the mouth for lipstick lines, carefully placed to avoid the corner of the mouth where smile muscles and the muscles used for chewing are present.

We still don't know the long term effects of Botox® treatment on the muscles, but it has been in clinical use since 1978 and no adverse long-term effects have been reported in the past 26 years. Recent widely-publicized stories of complications in Florida were misleading. The individuals involved did not use Botox® but rather an unapproved solution, manufactured in a laboratory. Please re-read the first section of this chapter and Chapter 10 about the importance of finding a board-certified, ethical doctor for your facial rejuvenation treatments.

## FILLERS

As we learned in Chapter 2, facial wrinkles and lines, other than lines of facial expression, are formed when our skin loses collagen and subcutaneous fat and the skin loses its elasticity and becomes lax. One solution is to inject a filler substance such as collagen into the deeper layer of the skin, the dermis, to plump up the depression or wrinkle. There are a wide variety of excellent fillers available today. There are so many products available, and they are so aggressively marketed, that it can be very confusing for you to know which filler, if any, is most suitable for you. You must rely on the knowledge of your physician. Thus, it is important to find a doctor who is knowledgeable about all of the fillers that are available. In my experience, each of the various types of filler has a specific application which is best done with that particular filler. The proper filler expertly placed in the appropriate patient produces a pleasing result (Figure 7-6).

Fillers are very popular and there are many new exciting types of filler available today. However, there

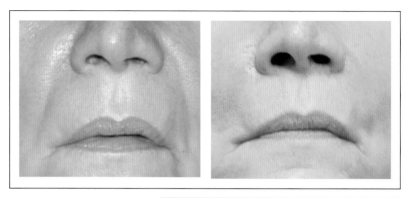

**FIGURE 7-6.**

*Before (left) and after (right) Radiesse®
injection into the nasal-labial fold lines.*

are two things you should keep in mind when you consider fillers.

First, fillers are a camouflage. They make the
wrinkle or line less noticeable, but they do nothing to
correct the basic problem. The problem that caused
the wrinkle in the first place – loss of collagen, elastin,
and subcutaneous fat, and the action of the facial muscles pulling on the skin for many years – is still present
and is not corrected by the injection of a filler.

For example, in the case of the nasal-labial fold
line (See Chapter 1), we plump the line by injecting

filler deep into the dermis underneath the line, which plumps the skin and makes the line less noticeable. The line is less noticeable, but the line is still present, and still caused by the overhanging, sagging cheek. A more corrective procedure would be to pull the cheek up and tighten it. That would be a face-lift. However many patients do not want to undergo a surgical procedure, preferring to have an improvement in the facial aging change rather than a surgical correction. For these patients fillers are an excellent alternative (Figure 7-7).

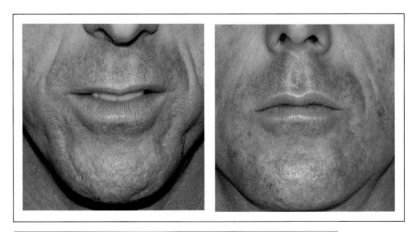

## FIGURE 7-7.

*Nasal-labial fold line, cheek wrinkle, and chin creases before (left) and after (right) Restylane® injection.*

Secondly, most fillers are temporary. Since fillers are foreign protein derived from animal sources (cow, pig, rooster comb), the body recognizes them as foreign proteins and degrades and removes them, in some cases as soon as three weeks! More permanent fillers are available, but there are risks. Silicone, one of the first fillers used, is a permanent filler, but it is not FDA approved because there is a high risk of complications, called granulomas. These are nasty, permanent bumps in your skin which can open, become infected, and drain. We'll stick with our discussion of safer, FDA-approved filler substances.

## Collagen – Zyderm®, Zyderm I®, Zyplast®

Collagen has been the most widely-used filler in the United States for more than 20 years. Zyplast® is the most popular form of collagen in use today. Zyplast® has been chemically altered to be less allergenic (less likely to cause an allergic reaction). It also lasts longer than earlier forms. It is injected into the dermis to plump up the skin and can be used to treat lines, scars and other depressions.

There are two main problems with collagen. The first is that roughly 3% of people are allergic to collagen and the allergy shows up as a nasty red bump. A simple skin test similar to a TB test is done on your arm to see if you are allergic to collagen. You must wait four weeks to see if your test is positive. A positive skin test would mean that you are allergic to collagen. Only after four weeks and a negative skin test can you then receive a collagen injection. The second drawback with collagen is that it does not last very long. It usually lasts no longer than three months.

There are many advantages to collagen. Collagen products contain an anesthetic which makes injection less painful. It is also less expensive per cc than the newer fillers, costing approximately $600 for a syringe which contains 2.75 ccs. I like the fact that I have much more volume when using Zyplast® and can easily treat several areas of the face.

# Hyaluronic Acid (HA) – Restylane®, Perlane®, Hylaform®

Do not confuse injectable Hyaluronic Acid (HA) which is a filler, with the HA creams we discussed in the last chapter. The creams are just moisturizers. Also, HA the filler is temporary and is used for its plumping action on the skin. Injectable HA has no magical anti-aging effects on your skin.

HA is a newer filler with several advantages over collagen. First, allergy to HA is not an issue, so skin testing is not required. Early studies indicate that HA may last longer than collagen, possibly up to six to eight months, another distinct advantage.

HA is marketed as Restylane®, Restylane Fine Lines® and Perlane®, and Hylaform®. They are all HA. It's just the size of the HA particles that varies. Restylane Fine Lines® has the smallest particle size and is placed high in the superficial dermis to treat fine lines. Restylane® has larger particles and is placed in

the mid dermis to treat moderately deep nasal-labial
fold line lines and in lip rejuvenation to plump up the lip
(Figure 7-8). Perlane® has the largest particle and is
placed in the deep dermis or subcutaneous fat to correct deep folds and to do facial contouring in patients
with sunken cheeks.

Unlike collagen, HA does not contain an anesthetic. Therefore, I use a topical anesthetic to numb the
skin first or alternatively use nerve blocks (like the
dentist), although that is rarely necessary. The
Restylane® fillers consist of HA, biologically-engi-

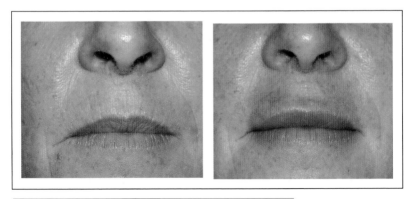

**FIGURE 7-8.**
*Lips, before (left) and after (right) Restylane®
injection. Note the lip is fuller, and the lipstick
lines are less noticeable after the filler injection.*

neered from bacteria. It is a mucopolysaccharide, not a protein like collagen, so is it less likely to produce an allergic reaction. Hylaform® is made from rooster comb.

HA treatments cost about $600 per syringe, but a syringe only contains about 1 cc which is approximately a third of the volume of a syringe of Zyplast®. One syringe of HA can usually treat the lips and mild or superficial nasal-labial fold lines. Deeper nasal-labial fold lines require two syringes and cost $1,000 to $1,200. It's high tech, but it's expensive.

## "Permanent" or Long Lasting Fillers – Radiesse®, Artefill®, and Sculptra®

Radiesse®, Artefill®, and Sculptra® are new fillers that are marketed as long-lasting or permanent fillers. They are not permanent! These ingeniously conceived, high tech fillers are also injected with a needle. Once injected, they stimulate your body to form your own tissue around the filler, producing a long-lasting result. Radiesse® uses calcium hydroxy apatite, a substance originally used to stimulate the body to make new bone. It has been modified, so that it absorbs water and forms a soft, viscous collagenous material beneath your skin which plumps up the line or defect and reportedly stays in place for one year. These fillers do not contain an anesthetic.

Artefill® uses polymethyl methacrylate (PMMA) spheres suspended in collagen. Over a three-month period after an injection, your own collagen grows in around the spheres resulting in a "permanent" fill. Sculptra® is the latest filler, made of poly L lactic acid, a substance that has been used for many years as suture material.

Sculptra® is quite different from Radiesse® and Artefill® in that it comes in a powder form which must be diluted with saline and lidocaine, an anesthetic. Also, the treatments must be repeated one or two times to get a final fill. Once it is in place, it is long-lasting, but it is more complicated to use than Radiance® and Artefill®.

The main problem with long-lasting or permanent fillers is we don't know what the long term (10-15 years), effect is going to be. They have been used for the past two to five years, especially in Europe and have been successful and safe enough to gain FDA approval. The honest answer is, we don't know if there are going to be long-term negative effects.

Permanent fillers must be injected into the mid dermis or deeper. Superficial injection can produce bumps called granulomas. Also, they are not FDA approved for use in the lips because of the risk of granulomas. I always insist that the patients try the non-permanent fillers, like collagen or HA first, to see if they like the effect. If a patient is happy with temporary fillers and is fully aware of the uncertainty and the potential long-term risks of more permanent fillers, I will then consider using the long-term filler. Long-term fillers are the most expensive at about $900 per treatment although prices are coming down as a result of competition from the HA fillers. I do like the way Radiesse® fills the nasal-labial fold line.

## THE ULTIMATE FILLER –
## YOUR OWN FAT

Your own fat can be harvested (removed) from an area of your body that doesn't need it (such as your hips) and injected back into your face to treat nasal-labial fold lines, puff up the lips and fill the tear trough deformity. Fat from your own body has the advantage of not being a foreign substance, so you don't need to worry about an allergic reaction.

Fat transplantation is a somewhat complex technique. Only about 35-50% of transplanted fat cells survive the process. So, most surgeons attempt to over-correct. In other words, they transplant 35-50% more fat than needed for the desired correction, allowing for shrinkage due to loss of the fat cells that don't survive the transplantation process.

Why don't we use this technique more often? Because it is surgery. It requires skill and training and you have to go through a two – to three – week recovery period during which you will be very swollen and bruised. Thus, it is not a "*no down time*" technique. However, if you don't want to bother with repeated filler injections, you don't mind the recovery period and you can find a surgeon skilled in this technique, fat transplantation can be a very beneficial treatment. It is most commonly done for nasal-labial fold lines, lip enhancement, and to correct the tear trough deformity. Fat injection around the eyes for the tear trough deformity is very tricky, though. Personally, I prefer blepharoplasty with muscle repositioning (See Chapter 8).

## CAUTION ABOUT FILLERS

The results or benefits you will see after the injection of any filler, whether it's collagen, Restylane®, Radiesse®, or fat, are *only as good as the skill of the person who injects these substances into your face.* The injection of a filler requires skill, expertise, and experience. It looks so simple on the videotapes that the filler companies give to your doctor as marketing tools. It is not simple. I have been doing it for 23 years and I still don't get it perfect every time. An inexperienced physician can easily push all the filler into the subcutaneous fat, which will have no effect on the wrinkle. Alternatively, it can be placed too superficially, just under the skin or epithelium, where it can cause a noticeable bump, or worse, a granuloma.

This is not something you want the occasional user to do to your face! Ask your doctor the right questions: How often does he or she do this? Are they experienced? Ask your friends how satisfied they were with the experience they had with this doctor. The thought of a nurse or non-physician doing a filler injection simply horrifies me!

## REFERENCES

1. Rubin, M. and Greenbaum, S. S. Histologic effects of aluminum oxide microabrasion on facial skin, J. Aesth. Dermatol. And Cos. Surg. 1: 237, 2000.
2. Shim, E.K., Barnette, D., Hughes, K. Et al. Microdermabrasion: A clinical and histopathologic study. Dermatol. Surg. 27: 534, 2001.
3. Tan, M., Spencer, J. M., Pires, L. M. The evaluation of aluminum oxide crystal microdermabrasion for photo-damage. Dermatol. Surg. 27: 943, 2001.
4. Brown, L.H., and Brancaccio, R. R. Injecting Botox: Tips from a master. Skin & Aging 10: 38, 2002.

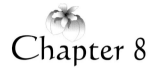

# Chapter 8

# HIGH-TECH FACIAL REJUVENATION:

### Lasers, Intense Pulsed Light (IPL), Infrared Light (Titan®), Radiofrequency (Thermage®), and LED (GentleWaves®) – Non-Ablative Therapies

Hold on to your pocket books. When you move up from vitamins, meditation, sun block, microdermabrasion, and Retin A you are going to start spending some serious cash. Before you do let me educate you as to the <u>truth</u> about these new and very tempting therapies.

One major problem you have is that the companies that make these machines have spent millions of dollars not only developing them and making them but also marketing them. Before the doctors are sure that they work as promised, the companies already have advertised them in the glamour magazines and have had testimonials on the TV talk shows. The result is that you show up in the doctor's office demanding the treatment and the doctor is backed into the corner – either buy the machine or lose you as a patient. It is a very unhealthy situation for you and the doctor. I urge you to study this chapter carefully.

I will teach you how these machines work, what they can do for you, what they cannot do for you, and more importantly how they can hurt you if they are not used correctly. Then you will be empowered to make a good choice.

Some of these machines can do wonderful and remarkable things to reverse aging changes in your face when used by qualified physicians who are up to date in their knowledge about the various modalities and machines. But you need to be able to wade through the hyperbole and find what you need and find the appropriate doctor to advise you. There is more on finding the right doctor in Chapter 10-Don't Let Just Anyone Touch Your Face.

## WHAT ARE HIGH-TECH "NON-ABLATIVE" THERAPIES?

To ablate as used here means to surgically remove. Non-ablative is used in this chapter to describe laser, IPL, radiofrequency, infrared light, and LED therapies. The machines used in these therapies do their work on your skin to remove pigment, blood vessels, and stimulate new collagen production *without surgically removing or damaging the top layer or epithelium of your skin.* The benefit of course is that if the skin is not ablated you will not have the long recovery time associated with ablative laser resurfacing and there will be less risk of scarring.

This is a very sophisticated highly technical process. These therapies are called non-ablative to distinguish them from the ablative procedure called laser resurfacing which is done with the more powerful $CO_2$ and Erbium lasers, both of which will be discussed in Chapter 8 under plastic surgical procedures. Do not be misled. These machines which are used for non-ablative therapies are powerful enough to cause ablation (removal) of your skin if they are not used properly by someone who is expert and skilled in their use. In my practice trained nurses under my supervision do some of these therapies.

Notice I said under my supervision, which means I am present on site at the time the treatments are done. I know that in many states it is legal for some of these therapies to be done at a spa or laser center by a nurse or technician when the "medical director", the doctor is not on site. In my opinion, this is far too dangerous and is unacceptable. I have seen some terrible complications following supposedly non-ablative laser procedures done by non-medically trained personnel in salons and spas.

Non-ablative facial rejuvenation procedures, when done for the right indication by a qualified person in a doctor's office, are effective and safe and eliminate much of the "down time" associated with traditional ablative procedures done in the past.

# NON-ABLATIVE LASER AND IPL FACIAL REJUVENATION

Be very careful here. These services are marketed to you as facial rejuvenation. That can be misleading. All reputable doctors agree that these techniques do a great job removing Type I facial aging changes such as brown spots and telangiectasias, but most will tell you these procedures *do not remove wrinkles and tighten skin*, the Type II facial aging changes. So do not be misled. Non-ablative laser and IPL therapy is very effective for:

- Removal of brown spots (pigment)
- Removal of telangiectasias (blood vessels around the nose, on the cheeks and chin)
- Removal of hair

## WHAT ABOUT WRINKLE REMOVAL?

While effective and safe non-ablative therapies have been available to treat brown spots, telangiectasias, hair, and tattoos for several years, the technology for wrinkle removal is still new and not nearly as effective and reliable as the other therapies. While some non-ablative laser treatments can stimulate new collagen production and slightly improve skin texture and wrinkles, the results are seen only after repeated treatments and after five to seven months. I want to help you understand how these therapies are supposed to work and what they can and cannot do for you.

## How Do Non-Ablative Laser and IPL Work?

Remember, in Chapter 2 I told you that the ultimate goal of all facial rejuvenation treatments is to remove pigment (brown spots), telangiectasias (blood vessels) and to restore the old, damaged collagen and elastin which have caused the skin to lose its elasticity and wrinkle. In previous chapters we have discussed how topical agents, exfoliation, Botox® and fillers attempt to accomplish the correction of these aging changes. Lasers and IPL (Intense Pulsed Light) attempt to correct aging changes in a very different high-tech way.

A phenomenal characteristic of lasers and IPL is that these machines can be manufactured to produce a very powerful beam of light that will only attack or destroy a specifically-colored target. This phenomenon is called **target specific photothermolysis**. Photothermolysis is light, heating and destroying a tissue such as pigment, a blood vessel, a cell, or collagen and elastin in your skin. The key phrase here is target specific. Unlike a shotgun, bomb or other high-powered form of energy, which destroy everything they hit, a laser or IPL can be tuned or controlled to damage only a tiny target of a specific color and not injure anything else in the surrounding area. For example, if you want to remove pigment use a laser or IPL light beam tuned to target only brown pigment. If you want to remove telangiectasias, you use a laser or IPL tuned to target only the red color of the blood inside a blood vessel.

This is possible because a laser or IPL beam is a light beam, an incredibly powerful, high – energy light beam (so powerful, a message can be sent to outer space on the back of a laser beam), which consists of only one color. The type of gas in the laser tube that is made to generate the laser beam, or the color of a lens in the IPL machine determines the color of the light beam that comes out of the machine. This characteristic allows us to target the light beam to one specifically – colored target – a red blood vessel, or a brown spot, or a blue tattoo.

Once the properly-colored light beam reaches the appropriate target, the high energy of the light beam (laser beam or IPL light beam) which is very hot, is absorbed by the specifically colored target. It heats the target and then ruptures or kills the target but does not damage the overlying skin. Thus if you want to remove a brown spot from the skin, you use a laser tuned to be absorbed by brown pigment. The skin is cooled as the laser passes through the epidermis into the pigment where the laser heat breaks up the pigment. Since the epidermis is not injured, there is no scar left behind. So, if you want to destroy something blue in the skin (a tattoo), you shine a powerful laser or IPL light beam tuned only to target blue in the skin. The laser will pass through the non-blue skin and be

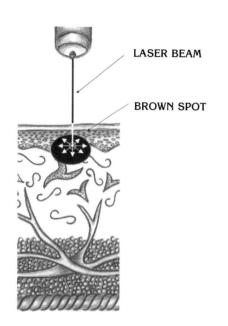

LASER BEAM

BROWN SPOT

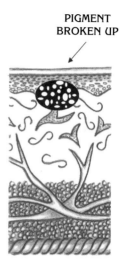

PIGMENT
BROKEN UP

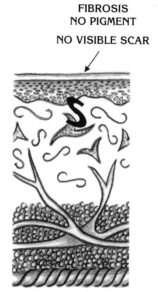

FIBROSIS
NO PIGMENT

NO VISIBLE SCAR

**FIGURE 8-1.**

*(Top Left) A laser
beam attacks a
brown spot. (Top
Right) Pigment is
broken up. Bottom)
Pigment is gone and,
after healing, there is
no visible scar.*

absorbed by, and thus destroy, the blue tattoo pigment. Practical application of the concept of target-specific photothermolysis was first applied on a clinically useful basis in the skin. Tattoo removal was the first; blood vessel and brown spot removal were next, and then came hair removal.

## NON-ABLATIVE WRINKLE REMOVAL?

Scientists have been trying for years to perfect this technique to target age-damaged collagen and elastin in the dermis (the deep layer of the skin), without damaging the epidermis (top layer) of the skin as the beam passes through on its way to the dermis. If this can be accomplished, the damage to the collagen and elastin caused by the laser or IPL beam causes inflammation, which you might remember from Chapter 3 is a process that results in fibrosis. Fibrosis is new collagen, produced in the wounded area by fibroblasts, the collagen producing cells which come into the dermis after inflammation. Yes, it is a scar, but a controlled scar. (See Chapter 3).

The theory is that if we can cause fibrosis in the dermis *without* injuring the overlying epidermis then the new collagen should restore elasticity, plump the skin, remove wrinkles, and tighten skin.

We are close, but the technique for wrinkle removal is not as effective as it is for removal of tattoos, blood vessels, brown spots and hair. Although this concept is theoretically possible, and the newer technology can produce microscopic new collagen regeneration, so far new collagen has been formed only in tiny, barely noticeable amounts. The best results show a 10% to 20% improvement in skin wrinkling, but honestly it is very hard to notice in the before and after photos.

More importantly, even though we call these therapies non-ablative, there is some risk of injury. As the laser beam passes through the outer layer of the skin, some of the heat energy heats the skin even though the outer skin is not the target. Potentially, the skin could be burned.

To avoid blistering the epidermis or outer skin, all lasers and IPL machines used for non-ablative therapies have some sort of cooling device to cool the skin during the treatment so that the hot laser or light beam passing through the skin does not heat and burn (blister) the skin on its way through the epidermis to the dermis. All of these machines have the power to burn your skin and create scarring if they are not used properly or if their skin cooling systems fail. It has happened. I have seen it with my own eyes.

If these machines do not remove wrinkles, then why in blazes then did I drag you through this tedious theoretical discussion? Because soon, probably before I finish my next book these non-ablative therapies will be improved to a point where they will work. I want you to understand how they work so you can ask the right questions and pick the right laser when that time comes. Check my website www.saveyourface.com occasionally and I will keep you updated. You will be the first to know when I know, I promise!

The particular name brand of the laser or IPL is less important than the expertise of the doctor you choose, so see Chapter 10 and learn how to choose the right doctor and trust him or her to know which laser or IPL is the best one for your treatment.

## INFRARED LIGHT (TITAN®) AND RADIOFREQUENCY (THERMAGE®) — NON-ABLATIVE SKIN TIGHTENING — THE "NON-SURGICAL FACE-LIFT"

The latest generation of infrared light and radiofrequency machines, Titan® and Thermage®, work very differently than lasers and IPL. Their potential usefulness is based on the fact that, when heated to 63 degrees centigrade, collagen shortens or tightens and "remodels." In other words, it is transformed into a new shortened or tightened form. When the collagen in the dermis of the skin treated by these machines is tightened, the skin is tightened. These machines produce "controlled" deeper heating over a larger area than the intense focused heating produced by a laser. These machines also use a very sophisticated cooling system to protect the overlying epidermis as the radiofrequency or ultraviolet light energy is passed through the epidermis (Figure 8-2).

## COOLING PHASE

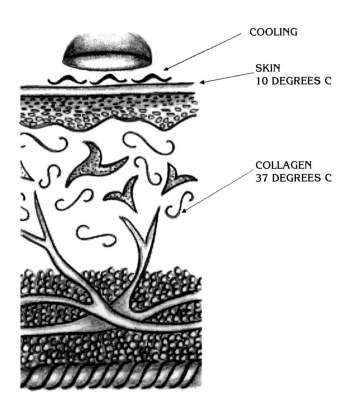

COOLING

SKIN
10 DEGREES C

COLLAGEN
37 DEGREES C

## FIGURE 8-2. A.)

*The skin is cooled prior to passing infrared or radiofrequency energy through the epidermis to heat the dermis.*

## COOLING AND HEATING PHASE

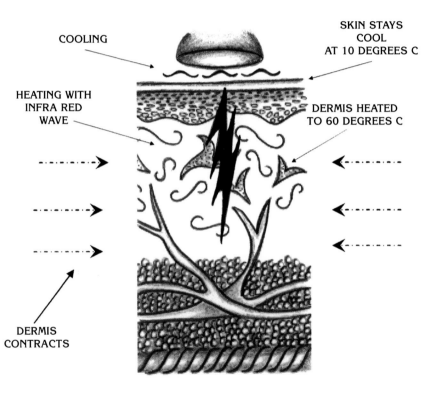

COOLING

SKIN STAYS
COOL
AT 10 DEGREES C

HEATING WITH
INFRA RED
WAVE

DERMIS HEATED
TO 60 DEGREES C

DERMIS
CONTRACTS

### FIGURE 8-2. B.)

*The skin cooled and energy is passed simultaneously into the dermis to heat the collagen in the dermis to 63 degrees centigrade.*

# COOLING PHASE

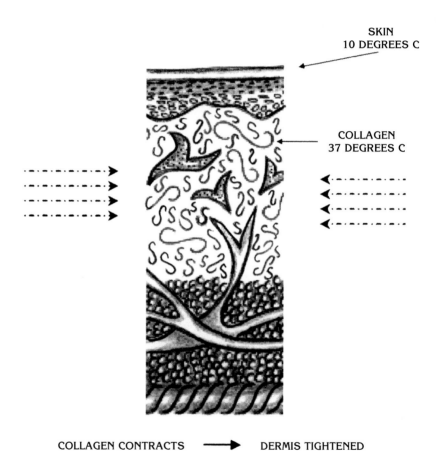

SKIN
10 DEGREES C

COLLAGEN
37 DEGREES C

COLLAGEN CONTRACTS ⟶ DERMIS TIGHTENED

---

## FIGURE 8-2. C.)

*The heated collagen shortens, skin is tightened, and the epidermis is not injured. Tightening of the skin can take 3 treatments over 3 to 5 months.*

The photographs of patients treated so far with the Titan® and Thermage® devices have been impressive when the procedure has been done on very thin skinned patients with virtually no fat underneath their skin. The manufacturers report on average a 30% tightening of the skin.

It takes at least three treatments, scheduled several weeks apart, to obtain a result. The final result will not be apparent for several months, the time it takes for the collagen to remodel. Although some patients see a result immediately, usually it takes three to five months for the final results to appear. This requires patience on the part of the patient, but this new therapy may be a good alternative for those not wanting surgery. Treatments cost $3500 to $5000 for a full series. The cost is determined by the size and difficulty of the area to be treated.

One drawback of this exciting non-ablative therapy is that it is a slow, tedious process, often taking an hour to do an entire face. Trained nurses and PAs under the supervision of the doctor can also do the actual treatment. Complications have been reported with Thermage®, most noticeably depressions or irregularity in the skin of the cheek and the side of the forehead, near the temple. Accordingly current guidelines recommend not treating those two areas. I do not see that as much of a problem. The areas we can treat – the jowls, neck, turkey wattle, chin, mouth, nasal-labial fold line, and forehead – are the areas where aging changes are most profound. Titan® is newer and, to date, I have not heard of complications with this machine.

Not all patients respond to these therapies. I assure you that within a year or so, we will know how to more accurately predict who will and who will not get a good result, how to avoid complications, and how to do a more effective treatment. I suggest you wait a few months and, in the meantime, use the proven therapies outlined in this book. You will make progress in your anti-aging battle and, who knows? The preparatory work you do may enhance the result you get from a high-tech skin tightening procedure in the future. Also, by next year, there may well be a newer, more effective non-ablative therapy. In fact, I can almost guarantee it.

I will keep you posted on my website, www.saveyour face.com.

# LED — (GentleWaves®)

LED stands for light emitting diode. LEDs are those little red lights that blink when you press the remote control for your TV set. You also see them on your microwave and other appliances. Why would any-one think of using them to treat facial aging?

According to the people who sell Gentlewaves® a scientist in the US space program was studying LEDs because, I assume, our astronauts are frequently exposed to a lot of LEDs during space flight. Fibroblasts growing in culture in a laboratory were exposed to LEDs and scientists discovered they made more collagen when they were exposed to LEDs than when they were not. If LEDs can stimulate collagen production by fibroblasts in the laboratory, then LEDs might be able to do the same thing in human skin. Right? Studies reveal some evidence to suggest that this concept is possible.

While clinical results were not as dramatic as they were with other non-ablative therapies, the LED treatments are very simple, safe, painless, and brief. Five seconds is all a treatment requires, and the patient feels nothing. The skin does not tighten and wrinkles do not disappear. However, Type I aging skin changes, brown spots, pigment, telangiectasias, rosacea, and skin texture are all reported to be improved after five weeks of one five-second treatment per week. The improvement is not as dramatic as it is with the laser and IPL.

This treatment is new, and long-term controlled studies of effectiveness are not completed, so the jury is still out on this therapy. But preliminary results are encouraging, especially considering the simple, safe, painless, quick nature of this treatment. It also costs about the same as a "face-lift in a jar" or a "better than Botox®", $100 to $125. It is definitely quicker, probably more fun, and you will be examined by a physician before the treatment. Hopefully he or she will also prescribe a retinoid or other proven effective skin preparation. When I know more about LEDs and their effectiveness, I will alert you on my website www.saveyourface.com.

After this lengthy technical discussion, what can non-ablative therapies do for you today? A great deal! These therapies can:

- Effectively and quickly correct Type I facial aging changes, such as brown spots, telangiectasias, and rosacea and remove unwanted hair without the scarring associated with traditional surgical methods of removal.
- With multiple treatments, over a period of several months, skin texture and minor wrinkling can be improved.
- Tighten the skin (of some of you) by about 30% especially in very thin individuals with very little subcutaneous fat.

These are dramatic and exciting new weapons in the anti-aging arsenal. Yes, they are more expensive than the "face-lift in a jar" and "better than Botox®" but these therapies actually work and in the long run, will probably save you money.

More importantly, when these therapies are combined with the "no down time" treatments discussed in

Chapter 7, and prescription skin creams listed in Chapter 6, you will definitely see visible gratifying reversal of Type I facial aging changes when you look in the mirror! If you also make the dietary, supplement, and lifestyle changes discussed in Chapter 4, you will amplify these exciting results, you will feel much better, and probably will live longer! Who could ask for more?

| AGING CHANGE | NON-ABLATIVE LASERS | IPL | LED | TITAN® THERM-AGE® |
|---|---|---|---|---|
| Remove pigment | yes | yes | slowly | no |
| Remove blood vessels | yes | yes | slowly | no |
| Improve skin texture | slowly | slowly | slowly | no |
| Remove fine wrinkles | slowly | slowly | ? | no |
| Tighten skin | no | no | no | Yes, slowly in thin individuals |

**TABLE 8-1.**
*What non-ablative therapies can and cannot do.*

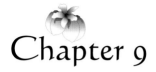

# Chapter 9

# WHAT CAN PLASTIC SURGERY DO FOR YOU?

Modern, properly-executed plastic surgery operations can beautifully and dramatically restore the aged human face to a much younger appearance. Plastic surgery can often make the face of a person look 20 or 30 years younger than their chronological age.

I have placed my discussion of plastic surgery at the end of this book, which is where it should be. All surgeons are taught to practice under the principle that surgery is the last option. Surgery is only to be considered when:

- All non-surgical medical therapies have failed.
- No medical therapies exist which can produce as effective a result or cure as surgery.

In this book, I have tried to educate you about most of the newer non-surgical treatments. Having done so, I now feel free to tell you about the surgical options. Cosmetic plastic surgery is elective, so the decision to have surgery must ultimately be reached by you. The decision as to when the more minor non-surgical options have failed is often a subjective one and requires sound, honest advice from your plastic surgeon.

Plastic surgery as a specialty has undergone a revolutionary and exciting transformation during my 23 years in this field. Research, education and continued improvement and refinement of anti-aging techniques are rigorously pursued by plastic surgery societies and all reputable plastic surgeons. The result is that, as of this writing, the surgical techniques available for reversal of facial aging are better, more effective, and safer than I would have believed possible when I was in training 25 years ago. So, if you are contemplating plastic surgery, let me assure you that the surgical procedures available to you are as technologically advanced and exciting as the antioxidant, holistic and non-ablative therapies I discussed earlier in this book.

Since the purpose of this book is to inform you about the available options to rejuvenate your face (and not a textbook to teach you how to perform plastic surgery), I will only briefly and generally discuss the more common facial rejuvenation procedures. These operations can truly rejuvenate your face and can give you a remarkable, lasting and beautiful result, if your expectations as a patient are realistic and if the procedure is performed by a competent plastic surgeon.

You notice I said patient. You are a "client" when you buy lipstick or skinceuticals. The minute a doctor touches you, you are a "patient." Don't forget it and always insist on it please!

## LASER RESURFACING

Laser resurfacing of the face is one of the most revolutionary new procedures for reversing facial aging to occur in the past 25 years. The ablative $CO_2$ and Erbium lasers can remove wrinkles, tighten skin and easily make your face look decades younger. But don't be fooled: Laser resurfacing is surgery. Laser resurfacing creates a wound on your face. When a wound is created, you have had surgery.

In Chapter 2, you learned how aging damage to the epithelium and collagen of your facial skin results in wrinkles and other aging changes. I told you that all anti-aging therapies attempt to make your skin new by stimulating the production of new epithelial cells and collagen. That is exactly what laser resurfacing does, all at once, and very aggressively.

The laser strips off the old epithelium and partially removes and injures the old, damaged collagen and elastin in the dermis. As a result of this injury, macrophages migrate from the blood into the skin, remove the damaged tissue and convert to fibroblasts to create new collagen. New epithelial cells grow over the face and form a new, young-looking epidermis. After the face has fully healed, the facial skin is tighter, fresher-looking and wrinkle-free. The reason the introduction of laser resurfacing has been such a revolutionary and rapidly accepted new procedure in plastic surgery is that this technique enabled us to correct facial aging changes that a face lift could not correct. While a face lift could correct jowling and tighten loose skin, patients were often disappointed by the fact that their facial skin still had fine wrinkles and sun damage after the face-lift. The laser has solved this problem, and for many patients eliminated the need for a face lift. (Figure 9-1).

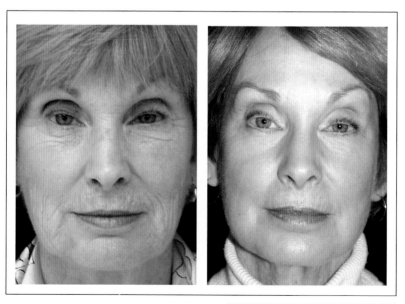

**FIGURE 9-1.**
*Before (left) and after (right) laser resurfacing.*

The photograph shows a patient before and after ablative laser resurfacing. When laser resurfacing is done correctly on the right person, the results are spectacular. Don't you agree?

But there is a catch. This is surgery, so you'll look terrible for ten to twelve days after surgery. You'll have to take meticulous care of your facial skin. In addition you'll be red to pink for at least six weeks, or longer, after surgery. Makeup will make you look fine after about two weeks, but don't even think about being seen in public without makeup for at least six weeks, possibly longer.

Fortunately with proper makeup you can go back to work and be seen socially by three weeks. It is crucial that the appropriate makeup be used. A special "mineral based" makeup created by Jane Iredale® is perfect for the patient who has had laser resurfacing. These superb makeups can also be used on normal skin.

The final, beautiful result is not complete until six months to a year after surgery, but you will be very happy even without makeup from three months on. Fair skin blondes and redheads with wrinkles and sun damage – that is people with Type I and Type II skin– cannot be given a fresher and younger-looking face by any other means including a face-lift.

Which laser? The $CO_2$ was the first laser to be used for laser facial resurfacing (1) and remains the "gold standard." However, I now use the Erbium laser made by Sciton®, the same scientific brainpower that invented the Ultrapulse® $CO_2$. The benefit of the Erbium laser is that it does not produce as much heat as the $CO_2$ laser does when the laser is used on your face. Less heat means less injury, and less injury means faster healing.

Generally, my patients who are treated with the Erbium laser heal in one-half to two-thirds the time it takes my $CO_2$ laser treated patients to heal. The Erbium laser-treated patients are less red for a shorter period of time and ready for makeup earlier. Long-term, there is less of a chance of hypo-pigmentation, which is whitening of the skin or lightening of the laser treated skin a year after surgery. There are still some situations in which the $CO_2$ laser is better than the Erbium laser. The decision as to which laser to use requires that your doctor be experienced in laser techniques.

Laser resurfacing is the best facial rejuvenation procedure for the right patient. The right patient has Type I or Type II skin with very severe wrinkles, sun damage and aging changes. NOTHING ELSE CAN DO AS GOOD A JOB!

Be sure your doctor shows you pictures of what you will look like three to four days and ten days after the operation. Also, the doctor needs to tell you about potential complications such as infection, scarring, hypo-pigmentation (whitening of the facial skin), prolonged redness, and potential eye injury. These things are rare, and should not happen to you, but they are real risks.

## FACE-LIFT

A properly done face-lift, technically called a rhytidectomy, can create an elegant, beautifully restored youthful facial appearance. The face-lift tightens facial skin and removes jowls, tightens the neck and removes the platysmal bands. The brow is elevated and the cheek and the malar fat pad are restored to their youthful position over the cheek bone. The nasallabial fold is tightened and, while the nasal-labial fold line does not disappear, the middle third of the face is freshened significantly. The jaw line is sculpted by a properly done face-lift and the tired sometimes angry look of the aged face is removed. Most commonly a face-lift is done in conjunction with a blepharoplasty or eyelid rejuvenation and the result is a nearly total facial rejuvenation that nothing else can match (Figure 9-2).

After looking at these pictures, do you REALLY BELIEVE you can look like that by simply slapping some antioxidant cream on your face? If pills and creams could really produce dramatic results like on the following page, then there would be photographs instead of case histories in the many books touting these therapies. So far, the photographs I have seen showing the results of topical creams and other non-surgical therapies are unimpressive.

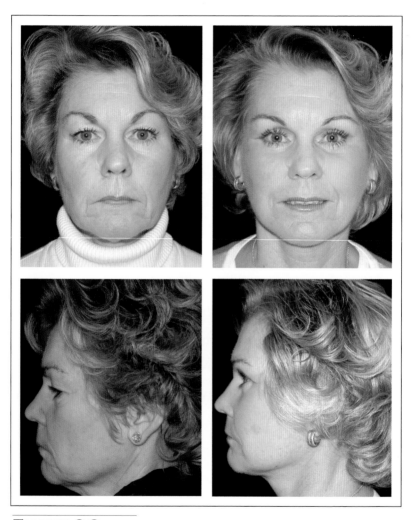

## FIGURE 9-2.

*Before (left) and
after (right) face-lift
and blepharoplasty.*

If a face-lift is what you need then have it, but have it performed by a properly-trained and board-certified plastic surgeon. (I will tell you in the next chapter how to find one.) What can a face-lift do? It can restore the firmness and integrity of your youthful face, remove jowls and sagging neck, lift the cheek, lift the brow and generally tighten the face. What can a face-lift not do? A face-lift can not freshen the surface of the skin, remove wrinkles and sun damage, brown spots, and dry, hard skin. For that, you need a laser resurfacing.

For many patients, the result of a face-lift can be dramatically improved by inserting a chin implant, which gives the patient a beautiful jaw line and youthful neck.

A face-lift firms or tightens loose, sagging facial skin. For fine wrinkles, pigmentation and sun damage, laser resurfacing must be done. Generally, face-lifting is more suited for darker skin types II, III, IV, V, and VI. Face-lifts are often helpful and often performed on patients with Type I or Type II facial skin with severe aging changes, but these patients usually need laser resurfacing, too, for the best possible result.

Your age at the time of your face-lift is your business. There are no hard and fast rules. When you see facial sagging in the cheek, the brow, the jaw, and the neck, and you are really bothered by these changes, seek a consultation with a reputable, board-certified plastic surgeon. It has been my experience that, with all restorative and maintenance endeavors, the earlier you repair something that is showing signs of age and wear, the better and longer-lasting the repair! I believe the same is true for the face.

A face-lift should not make your face look tight, pulled, or unnatural. A face-lift should make you look like you did when you were younger. If someone looks like a weasel, this means they either had a bad lift or have had one too many (face-lifts, that is!) Look again at the photos. These patients simply look younger, not different.

What can go wrong? Potentially, many things, is the short answer. Picking the right surgeon is the key to avoiding problems. Some problems are caused by a failure in your doctor's technique, some are failures in your anatomy and healing and some are, believe it or not, simply fate.

I show my patients photographs of what they will look like the first day, a few days later, and ten days to two weeks after surgery. I want them to have no surprises. Your surgeon should inform you of the possible complications. They are frightening, and they include: bleeding, infection, scarring, skin loss, hair loss, permanent paralysis of your face, loss of feeling in the face, asymmetry or differences in the right and left sides of your face, lumps, bumps, and recurrence of sagging. No one can guarantee you a result. Every patient heals differently. One goal is for your result to last ten to fifteen years, but some patients – generally those with severe sun damage and Type I skin – need a re-do face-lift after two years.

In the hands of a skilled, board-certified plastic surgeon, THESE COMPLICATIONS ARE VERY RARE. If they were not, we would not be allowed to do this operation. Who would want to? But they can happen and you need to be informed in advance.

Recovery from a face-lift is usually easier than that from a laser resurfacing. The first week after a face-lift you will be bruised and swollen although some patients have very little swelling or bruising. Most patients are in makeup by two weeks and back to work by three weeks at the latest.

Be wary of the highly marketed mini-face-lift or week-end tuck. Some patients with minimal facial aging changes get an acceptable result from these less extensive procedures. Many however show up in my office needing a revision after having the mini-procedure elsewhere. Of course the patient ends up paying twice for one final result. As always, it is crucial that you seek expert opinion from a credible source.

## BROW-LIFT

Since the advent of Botox®, which can help elevate the brow, brow lifting alone is becoming less common. Typically, I perform brow-lifting at the same time I do my face-lift. However, some patients need only a brow-lift. The brow-lift is done either through tiny scalp incisions with an endoscope or with incisions which are hidden in the hairline. Below is an example (Figure 9-3).

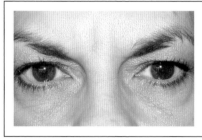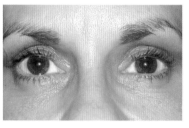

**FIGURE 9-3.**
*Before (left) and after (right) brow-lift and blepharoplasty.*

Complications can include numbness in the forehead, patches of hair loss and recurrence of sagging. Recurrence of brow sagging can and does happen in about a third of patients. Recovery is much quicker than from a face-lift, usually a week.

# EYELID REJUVENATION – BLEPHAROPLASTY

The eyes are truly the "windows of the soul" and of all our facial features, considered to be the most important. Studies have been done on infants who were shown only portions of their mother's face, chin, mouth, nose, forehead, and eyes. The one part of the face they most frequently and easily recognized was their mother's eyes.

Unfortunately, as I mentioned in Chapter 2, we age first in our eyes, most commonly in the 30s, and some of us in our late 20s. Eyelid rejuvenation is by far the most common and early plastic surgery operation I perform. The results are usually dramatic, pleasing and successful.

Blepharoplasty is intended to correct or partially correct the following aging changes:

- Hooding or hanging skin of the upper eyelid
- Puffiness (fat herniation of both upper and lower eyelids)

- Laxity or looseness of the lower eyelid
- Tear trough deformity (that line under the lower eyelid).

A blepharoplasty alone cannot correct:

- Brow sagging
- Eyelid wrinkles
- Aging damage to eyelid skin
- Crow's feet

Personally, I use the laser for my eyelid rejuvenation procedures. There is less bruising and quicker recovery. Also, I don't make an incision on the outside of the lower eyelid. I use the laser to make an incision on the inside of the lower eyelid, the pink part (transconjunctival blepharoplasty.) From the inside of the lower eyelid, I remove or reposition the fat to remove the bulge and partially correct the tear trough deformity. I also use the laser on the inside to shrink or tighten the underlying muscle. Following these maneuvers, I frequently do what is called a canthopexy. The canthopexy is a procedure done through the upper eyelid incision to tighten the tendon of the lower eyelid, re-creating the nice curved, upward slanting lower eyelid appearance of our youth.

I then do laser resurfacing on the skin of the lower eyelid to rejuvenate the appearance of the skin and remove crow's feet. What's the point of tightening the lower eyelids and removing the bags, if the patient still has sun damaged aged skin on the eyelid? Patients must go through a period of healing during which the lower eyelid is red, but when the eyelid has healed and the patient sees brand-new smooth skin on the eyelid, they are very happy. (Figure 9-4).

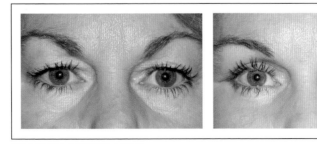

**FIGURE 9-4.**
*Before (left) and after
(right) laser
blepharoplasty.*

Eyelid wrinkles and crow's feet are also caused by the pulling of the muscle underneath the skin. Therefore, in my practice, I use Botox® to quiet the muscle after surgery and encourage the patient to continue to have Botox® treatment of the "crow's feet".

The laser is a marvelous, technologically-advanced tool that can create optimal results in eyelid rejuvenation. Not all surgeons are comfortable with or competent in the use of the laser. You should find a doctor experienced in and comfortable with the use of the laser.

Complications are rare, but you must be informed: Bleeding, infection, scarring, dry-eye syndrome (very serious), and ectropion, a sad-eyed or "hound dog appearance" more common with the external scalpel incision on the lower eyelid. (Just walk down Rodeo Drive or Fifth Avenue and you will see it!) Other complications include loss of eyelashes, damage to the eye or even blindness (1 in 800,000 operations). These complications are rare, but serious. Your surgeon needs to discuss them with you.

The above procedures are the most common and effective plastic surgical operations to correct facial aging. In the next chapter I will try to help you to make a very important decision if you are considering having plastic surgery.

## REFERENCES

1. Seckel, B. R. Aesthetic Laser Surgery, 1st Ed. Boston: Little, Brown and Company, 1995.

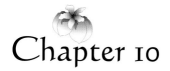

# Chapter 10

# DON'T LET
# "JUST ANYONE"
# TOUCH YOUR FACE!

I am astounded when I hear stories of people who have had potentially dangerous medical and surgical therapies performed by untrained uncertified people who are not doctors. Recently, in Massachusetts (where I live), home of the Harvard Medical School and many world famous doctors and hospitals, police raided a house in one of our suburbs where a man and his wife with no medical training whatsoever were performing blepharoplasty, eyelid surgery in their home.

I do not know what people are thinking when they subject themselves to such risks, but I do know what they are not thinking. They are not thinking about what they will do when something goes wrong such as an infection or bleeding. Nor are they thinking about what they will do if the procedure does not produce the result that they expect.

There are already significant worries that untrained people without appropriate skills are doing cosmetic facial rejuvenation procedures in this country (1). More frightening is the fact that there is a proliferation of retail centers called spas where nurses and other non-physicians are doing potentially dangerous procedures, supposedly under the supervision of physicians who are not even present at the facility!

I believe a major factor in these occurrences is the perception that cosmetic procedures are simpler than major surgery and therefore less dangerous. Adding to this misconception is the skill and ease with which properly trained physicians do these procedures, making them look deceptively easy to other physicians and nurses who watch them. In the western United States, a death occurred when a nurse opened her doctor's office at night and performed a liposuction on a friend without the doctor's knowledge. Her friend, the patient, died. I am sure the nurse had watched the doctor do the operation hundreds of times and thought it was simple. Unfortunately, the procedure, which looked so easy when the surgeon was doing it, required skill which can only be learned in a surgical residency. She accidentally shoved the suction cannula into her friend's liver and the friend bled to death. Do you need to hear more?

Many of the non-surgical procedures we perform, such as Botox® and filler injections, laser treatments, and microdermabrasions, are so quick and seemingly easy that you, the patient, do not have the same concern or caution that you would if you were considering surgery. The problem is, as always, what happens if something goes wrong? What if the Botox® or the filler is put in the wrong place? How do you set the power of the laser, and how many times do you treat the blood vessel or brown spot?

Money is what is driving these dangerous and misguided practices. The patient wants to spend less of it and the non-physician entrepreneurs performing these "back alley" procedures want to make more of it. Unfortunately, bad things always happen when greed overcomes judgment, principles, and ethics.

Hopefully, since you are mindful enough to read this book, you will find a qualified physician to advise you and provide or supervise your facial rejuvenation therapies. It is the uninformed people whom I worry about! So do your part and educate your friends.

So where do you go for advice and treatment for facial rejuvenation? In the United States today, most physicians specializing in facial anti-aging or facial rejuvenation are plastic surgeons and dermatologists. I am certain there are many others who, as a result of their training, interest and experience, are capable. But the board certification process in plastic surgery and dermatology provides educational standards that are widely recognized and upheld. Insisting on board certification in one of the above specialties is a good starting place for you, the consumer.

However, consulting a board-certified physician is just the beginning of the process. A certificate on the wall cannot tell you how skilled the doctor is and how expert he or she is in facial rejuvenation procedures. There is much more to making an informed decision, as follows.

## Be Careful — Your Fear is Your Friend — How to Pick Your Doctor

Everyone–and I mean everyone–who comes to see a plastic surgeon for the first time is uneasy or fearful. This is a normal self-protective response and you should heed it. Surgery, or any facial procedure, is a very serious undertaking. Essentially, you are giving another person, hopefully a doctor, control over your facial appearance, your well-being, and (in the case of surgery), even your life. This is not something you should take lightly and most people have inherent emotional, instinctual responses which "raise a red flag" when you contemplate giving up control of your well-being. In my experience, there are only two things that can help eliminate your fears especially when considering the possibility of surgery:

- Complete trust and confidence in your plastic surgeon

or

- Ignorance (Sorry for the harsh words, but this is IMPORTANT)

Obviously #2 does not apply to you or you wouldn't be reading this book.

Unfortunately, there are thousands of people who consider having plastic surgery with as much forethought as they do when they buy a loaf of bread or new blouse. These are the people you see on talk shows condemning plastic surgery because they did not get the results they wanted or worse, they have been injured. These are tragic but, fortunately, rare occurrences and, like most mistakes we make in life, they could have been avoided.

Fortunately, because you're a contemplative and intelligent person, you can do the requisite self-education about plastic surgery and learn what you need to know and how to choose a plastic surgeon whom you can trust to do it right. Knowledge and your "gut instinct" will lead you to the right person. Remember, 99% of unhappy results are avoidable.

## What is a Surgeon?

Believe it or not, in the United States today you cannot just assume that a doctor who calls himself a "surgeon" is a surgeon. I am sorry to tell you that some prominent M.D.s in major metropolitan areas of the United States who openly advertise themselves as "cosmetic surgeons" have never had one day of surgical training!

There are also many, certainly hundreds maybe even thousands of people who call themselves "plastic surgeons" who have never had one day of training in an approved plastic surgery residency!

How can this be? How has this happened in a country where the USDA protects our meat supply and the FDA helps keep harmful drugs out of our hands? (Ever heard of mad cow disease or Vioxx®?) The simple answer is twofold:

1. We live in a democracy. You can call yourself anything you like. The American Society of Plastic and Reconstructive Surgery tried, about twenty-five years ago, to protect you from this deception by attempting to prove in court, that if you called yourself a plastic surgeon, you should have board certification and training in plastic surgery. The courts ultimately ruled against the plastic surgery society with decision that stated that, to require certification in plastic surgery in order to call oneself a plastic surgeon was a "restraint of free trade" and violated the Federal Commerce and Communication Act. So much for standards and protections for you the consumer!

2. There is big money in plastic surgery. Managed care has made it very difficult to make a living in medicine today, let alone pay off the average $250,000 debt acquired during training in medicine. In this country, there is a widely held misperception that all

doctors are wealthy. In fact, most doctors who finished their training in 2005 can't even think about buying a house until they pay down the debt they acquired getting their education.

Aesthetic or cosmetic plastic surgery is the only "fee for service" or "cash and carry field" left in medicine and it can be very lucrative. Unfortunately, many doctors without formal training or board certification market themselves as "cosmetic surgeons" or "plastic surgeons" because they want to make money and they are not qualified or don't want to take the five – to seven – years of residency training after medical school that is required to become a fully-trained, board-eligible plastic surgeon.

So, dear reader, I have provided you with two of the most important reasons why you should be afraid of letting "just anyone" touch your unique face. It can be a snake pit out there in certain portions of the non-medical and medical community, and those of you who simply "let your fingers do the walking" in the yellow pages might as well buy your snake-bite kit and start taking anti-venom now.

In my 23 years as a plastic surgeon, I have seen some unfortunate complications of plastic surgery performed by unqualified people. When I asked the patient how they found the doctor, the most common answer, you guessed it, was the yellow pages! Another poignant memory is a woman with terrible scarring who told me, with embarrassment, that her maid had recommended the doctor! Think about it. Do you think the telephone companies ask "are you board certified?" before they take $5,000 to list someone's ad in their book as a plastic surgeon? I doubt it.

So if you can't trust the phone book, or your maid to help you, how do you find a well-trained, board certified plastic surgeon? Contact the American Society of Plastic Surgery at (888) 4-PLASTIC or their website www.plasticsurgery.org. You must be an experienced Board-Certified Plastic Surgeon to be listed with this organization. After you have done your homework and are armed with knowledge, you can start the interview process and evaluate your prospective plastic surgeon. After you have interviewed them, you will then have to listen to the most important protector you have, your gut instinct.

# What Is A Board Certified Plastic Surgeon?

The straightforward, honest answer, and the only answer you should accept, is: A doctor with an M.D. degree, who, after completing medical school, spent five to seven years in an accredited, (approved by the American Council on Graduate Medical Education/ACGME), residency training program in one or more fields of surgery, the last two years of which were spent in an approved Plastic Surgery Residency Training Program. The preliminary surgery part may be spent in General Surgery, Orthopaedic Surgery, Urology, Neurosurgery, Otolaryngology or other ACGME-approved surgical subspecialty but the last two years must be spent in an approved Plastic Surgery Residency Program.

After five to seven years of training, the doctor is still not a Board-Certified plastic surgeon. The doctor must then, over the next two years, successfully practice (frightening phrase!) plastic surgery, taking care of and operating on patients. During this period, they must pass a rigorous written examination to document that they have an adequate knowledge of the art and science of plastic surgery. Next, they must submit a list of all the plastic surgery operations they have performed in those two years to the American Board of Plastic Surgery and then undergo and pass a comprehensive and rigorous oral examination.

Prior to the examination, senior experienced Board Certified Plastic Surgeons called Board Examiners (I have been one of them, so I know of what I speak) scrutinize the candidate's list of operations for mistakes, bad judgment, unscrupulous billing and other inappropriate behavior before allowing the candidate to take the exam. Believe me when I tell you that after all this, some candidates are sent home and not allowed to finish the exam. It is very sad and a difficult thing to do, but it means that you, the patient, are the American Board of Plastic Surgery's primary concern. Your safety and the reputation of our specialty take precedence over anything else!

If the candidate is accepted into the examination, he or she then goes through two days of oral examinations in a series of four sessions by two senior Board Certified Plastic Surgeons with one candidate face-to-face. It is a no-holds-barred, complex examination to see if the young surgeon is fit in the eye of these senior surgeons to be called Board Certified in Plastic surgery. People still fail at this late point and are not allowed to call themselves board-certified plastic surgeons. Think about it – ten years of training and experience after medical school and you still have to pass the most rigorous personal scrutiny and testing by the senior most experienced surgeons in the field.

Is this the type of doctor you want to operate on your face? Of course it is. This type of information is not clearly available in the yellow pages or newspapers, on the radio or on TV talk shows, on billboards or on the Internet. It is, however, readily available to you, the educated consumer, by calling the American Board of Plastic Surgery (215-587-9322, www.abplsurg.org). That is how you start your search.

Dermatologists also have made great contributions to the science of facial aging and have been pioneers in the discovery of "skinceuticals", lasers, and many of the non-ablative skin treatments discussed earlier in this book. The huge advance in aging research and breakthroughs in the genetic modification necessary to reverse aging on the molecular level will probably be made, in part, by dermatologists. They are the skin doctors and they can do a great deal to help you in your anti-aging battle. However, they are not surgeons in the sense that they have not trained in surgical residencies as described earlier.

Most importantly, a fully trained surgeon is trained in how to take care of the whole patient, not just the skin or face, especially if something goes wrong. Furthermore, in my opinion, it takes the five to seven years of specialized training and experience to learn and understand the complex anatomy and aging changes that plastic surgery can correct.

**There is no American Council on Graduate Medical Education (ACGME) recognized surgical subspecialty designated as "cosmetic surgery." Caveat emptor!**

## Educate Yourself

If you are considering plastic surgery, your medical doctor should refer you to someone whom he or she knows is well-trained, ethical, and highly skilled. More commonly, happy patients who have had a positive experience with a particular plastic surgeon make plastic surgery "referrals." If, however, you do not have the benefit of either of those resources, call the sources listed above for a referral in your area. I recommend that you get the names of at least two board certified plastic surgeons.

You are, however, only halfway there. The surgeon you have selected will have to pass another test or oral examination to earn your trust and the privilege and honor of being your doctor.

I sincerely mean that it is an honor and a privilege for a surgeon to have you as a patient. My mentor, and the man who trained me as a plastic surgeon, was Dr. Joseph E. Murray, Chair of Plastic Surgery at Brigham and Women's Hospital in Boston,

Massachusetts and Professor of Surgery at Harvard Medical School. Dr. Murray won the Nobel Prize in Medicine for his work in performing the first kidney transplantation, an event that gave birth to the remarkable field of transplantation surgery. This field has grown to a level where now kidneys, hearts, lungs, livers, bowels and other essential organs are transplanted, saving lives and preventing disability for thousands of people.

A plastic surgeon started all this? Yes, indeed. Throughout my training and to this very day Dr. Murray (now in his eighties) still smiles, eyes glowing, and says, "I feel so privileged and honored to be able to be a surgeon," and he means it.

He is the greatest living plastic surgeon and he is honored and privileged to take care of you. Can anyone else be less so? You, the patient, are giving us a great honor and privilege by trusting us with your lives and well-being. Any surgeon who forgets that and views you as a down payment on a Ferrari or Lamborghini, deserves to be stripped of all credentials and sent packing. This doctor has violated your trust.

So what can you do to be as certain as possible the surgeon you have chosen is a person who has not only the education and skills to do a good safe face-lift or other procedure, but also has the ethical and moral constitution to give you his or her best? Unfortunately, board certification and credentials can't provide you with this insight. Only your instincts and intuition, your gut feelings, plus the insights and experiences of other patients who have been treated by the same doctor can help you there. So here's my advice, my recommendations for your consultation:

Do your homework. The American Society of Plastic Surgeons (888-4-PLASTIC, www.plasticsurgery.org) and the American Society of Aesthetic Plastic Surgeons (800-367-2147, www.asaps.com) provide easy to understand information about all cosmetic surgery. You can call them or go to their websites and receive educational brochures about any procedure you are interested in. Do this and read about the surgery you are considering.

Write down your questions ahead of your consultation. Be prepared. If you have knowledge, you have power. You must know what to ask your surgeon. Ask the right questions. Here are a few questions that may not be in the brochures:

1. Are you certified by the American Board of Plastic Surgery? Get a straight answer here, look on the wall. The certificate is unmistakable (Figure 10-1).

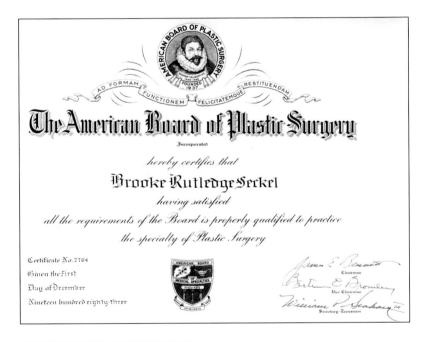

**FIGURE 10-1.**
*Board certification certificate for plastic surgery.*

2. Are you experienced in or do you specialize in aesthetic and cosmetic plastic surgery? This is important, I believe. Many superb Reconstructive Plastic Surgeons have little experience in Cosmetic Plastic Surgery. You must ask the question.

3. How many of these operations have you done? Do you do them frequently? (I mean weekly.)

4. Are you comfortable operating on me? Are you confident you can get a good result on my face, eyes, breast, or body? We are all very different with specific, challenging anatomical issues.

5. What can go wrong? What are the possible complications? How often do they happen?

6. What happens if something goes wrong? Is a revision or correction free of charge or will I have to pay for it?

7. How many visits or how many times after surgery do I get to see you? Can I reach you or someone

with access to you 24/7 after my surgery? Is someone available to see me nights, weekends, or holi-
days if I have a problem?

8. Will you allow me to contact and talk with patients
you have operated on who can tell me what their
experiences have been?

These are excellent questions to ask and you
have every right to expect clear, honest answers. They
reflect that you have done your homework and are an
educated patient. Believe me; a good surgeon will be
grateful that you are prepared.

Patients who are unprepared and lack knowledge become huge problems after surgery. I try very
hard to inform my patients of what to expect before
surgery. We give informed consent, in the form of legal-
ly-prepared documents, outlining possible complications and problems. Research has shown that the
patients forget 90% of what they are told and what they
have confirmed by their signatures that they have read
and understood.

This is a very difficult problem. It may be hard, but you, the patient need to do your part, and be an educated consumer.

## TRUST YOUR "GUT FEELINGS" AND "RED FLAGS" ("RUN FORREST, RUN!")

Here I am stating what should seem to be the obvious, but then, how many times in our lives do we have that gut feeling, ignore it, make a decision and regret it? Having plastic surgery is not like buying a car, an expensive diamond or a $10,000 gown. Those things can be a bad choice that costs you money and puts you in debt, but you are still alive and well afterwards! Your friends can still recognize you and you can learn from your mistake and restore your life.

Choosing the wrong person to do plastic surgery on your face could result in irreversible deformity, loss of your health or self-esteem, and turn your happiest dreams into a nightmare.

I don't want to dissuade you. Many thousands of people have superb plastic surgery every year in this country and complications are very, very rare when the right operation is done on the right patient by the right surgeon. I want the best for you and want you to have a good experience. If you do, you will bring happiness to yourself and honor to my profession. But there are a few things that I call red flags-warnings from your intuitive self that are trying to protect you. Listen to them:

• First, remind yourself that the doctor you are seeing wants you as a patient. Cosmetic surgery is elective surgery, and you are paying cash for your operation. You are doing the favor here. The doctor should be kind, warm, concerned and respectful of you as a person. If he or she doesn't make you feel this way, then smile politely, say, "Thank you, I will get back to you when I make my decision," and leave. The most important question to ask yourself is, "Do I trust this person? Will I feel comfortable having this person take care of me if something goes wrong?" If the answer is no, leave. Remember what Jenny said in the movie Forrest Gump? when the mean boys were chasing him she yelled, "Run, Forrest, Run".

- The surgeon is cold. This one should be a no-brainer. It's not your problem if the surgeon's parents weren't nurturing enough or if this person's life has been tough. Some of our greatest geniuses (think Mozart) are driven to achieve great skills by their tormented souls. Years of training, scrutiny and rigorous testing cannot guarantee basic human compassion and kindness. Trust your feelings. Talk to the doctor. Look in their eyes and face. Would you be comfortable asking this person to help you when you are frightened, in need, even with your silliest question? You should be. If you are not, "Run Forrest, Run!"

- The surgeon gets uncomfortable, defensive or angry when you ask those important questions that you must ask. Again, trust your instincts. He should welcome your questions and answer them to your satisfaction. If you see sweat on his or her brow or the initial warm glow of your meeting disappears, "Run, Forrest, Run!"

- The surgeon does not act like a doctor. Personally, I like a white coat or a conservative suit or dress.

Even casual relaxed is okay. I frequently wear scrubs and a white coat in my office. If your surgeon looks or acts like a used car salesman or looks like he or she is dressed to go onstage in Las Vegas, I would get nervous. The surgeon's professionalism and credentials are what is important here not the authentic Ming vase in the waiting room. Don't get me wrong. I love Ming vases (wish I could afford one) and pretty things. I believe and it is my practice in my office that the plastic surgery office should be appointed and designed for your comfort and enjoyment. But if you are more awed by the decor and the trappings than by the professionalism of the surgeon, "Run, Forrest, Run!"

- The surgeon or the staff makes you feel stupid for asking a question. Come on now, you wouldn't be reading this book if you didn't already know that game. Do you like or trust or want to be around anyone who makes you feel less than you truly are, which is a worthwhile human being with normal concerns, anxieties and fear? You are coming to a professional whose job it is to make you feel good about yourself. If you do not, "Run, Forrest, Run!"

- If it seems too good to be true, it is. C'mon, you know this. If this thought pops in your mind, respect it, "Run, Forrest, Run!"

- Plastic surgery is not cheap. Surgery includes the skills and training of your surgeon and very high tech, expensive equipment, anesthesia, nursing and complex postoperative care. Any plastic surgeon who offers you a cut-rate deal is leaving out something important and when it comes to your health and safety you cannot afford to leave anything out. The American Society for Aesthetic Plastic Surgery publishes average fees for various cosmetic procedures in this country. Simply ask your surgeon how his or her fee compares to the national average. Yes, it is cheaper in an office than a hospital, but is it a safe office? Ask where you are taken if something goes wrong. In plastic surgery, I would be less worried if a surgeon charges more than the average. There is usually a good reason. They are the best, and their expertise and reputation permit them to charge more. Whether they are really worth it can be ascertained when you speak with patients who have had operations performed by that surgeon. Be sure to ask for permission to talk with previous patients. If someone offers you a bargain or a cut rate, "Run Forrest, Run!"

- The plastic surgeon's staff-the receptionist, nurses, assistant, technicians, physician assistants, and medical aestheticians – all play a crucial role in your experience. They will be providing a significant role in your post-operative care and will be invaluable to you. Talk with them and trust your instincts. Are they professional, warm, kind, caring people you would be comfortable asking for help and depending on? Don't choose them because they are physically attractive, well dressed, starlets. They are healthcare professionals, not models. If you feel like you do not belong there, you most certainly do not. "Run Forrest, Run!"

- Choose a plastic surgeon who performs a lot of cosmetic surgery. Plastic surgery involves not only knowledge and judgment but, as surgery, requires manual skills and dexterity. Those who don't have it are typically weeded out during training. However, whether you are playing a piano, painting a house, doing a cross-stitch or performing plastic surgery, practice makes perfect. The American Society for Aesthetic Plastic Surgery (800-367-2147, www.-asaps.com) is a society of plastic surgeons who have a special interest in and expertise at cosmetic plastic surgery. Their website has detailed information about all cosmetic procedures and is an excellent place for you to learn about the procedure you are considering. Unequivocally, the surgeon who does facial cosmetic procedures every week will be better than the one who does them occasionally, every month or so. Ask the surgeon that question and gauge the response. If it makes you feel anxious, "Run Forrest, Run!"

Finally, in deference to my younger colleagues, let me say that old and experienced is not necessarily better than young and skilled. Gray hair is no guarantee. There are many brilliant, young board-certified plastic surgeons in this country who are better educated, trained and skilled than ever before. They can do as good, or even a better, job than an older less-talented surgeon. It's a balance. You need to ask the right questions and trust your instincts – your gut feelings. And remember, it is important to talk to prior patients.

## PLASTIC SURGERY ADDICTION – BODY DYSMORPHIC DISORDER

In my experience most patients seeking facial rejuvenation treatments and plastic surgery are sensitive, wonderful, sane, well adjusted individuals who consider looking their best one part of an over-all positive attitude toward life and health. There are however some people who seek plastic surgery not simply to fight aging and improve the way they look but rather to correct some imagined deformity that only they can see. This type of patient is more likely to be young and there is evidence that this phenomenon is more common in males.

All ethical, well-trained, board certified plastic surgeons should be aware of this disorder, called body dysmorphic disorder, and encourage these individuals to seek psychiatric care not surgery. However, as I mentioned earlier in this chapter there are many unscrupulous inadequately trained non-medical and medical practitioners in this country who are more concerned about making money than the health and welfare of the patient. Often, patients who have been turned down by reputable plastic surgeons end up having their surgery in these "back alley" practices frequently with disastrous results.

The media refers to people who have had too many plastic surgical procedures as "plastic surgery addicts". However the proper medical terminology for such individuals is body dysmorphic disorder. This is a serious, painful, distressing obsession with imagined physical deformity. When you see a person with this disorder you usually cannot imagine what they find unappealing about their appearance! Individuals afflicted with this illness go to incredible behavioral extremes to modify their appearance. I am not talking about 3 or 4 plastic surgeries but 10 or 20!

Obviously the doctor has to avoid operating on such an individual. However patients are not always honest and forthcoming about their medical history and it is possible for a well meaning physician to be misled and operate on such an individual without being fully aware of the patient's motivation for surgery.

Body dysmorphic disorder is defined (2) as follows:

- Preoccupation with some imagined defect in appearance. If a slight physical anomaly is present, the persons concern is markedly excessive.

- The preoccupation causes clinically significant distress or impairment in social, occupational, or other important areas of functioning.

- The preoccupation is not better accounted for by another mental disorder (e.g. dissatisfaction with body shape and size in anorexia nervosa).

The above definition does not describe an individual who is a "little vain", rather it characterizes an individual with a serious obsessive disorder. If the above description applies to you or someone you love, or a friend I urge you to read or refer the involved person to " The Broken Mirror " by Katherine A. Phillips, M.D. Help is also available at the Westwood Institute For Anxiety Disorders, Inc. (www.hope4ocd.com).

## KEEP UP-TO-DATE

The field of anti-aging medicine generally, and facial rejuvenation in particular, is advancing rapidly. New information and therapies are discovered almost daily. It is crucial that you continue to read and inform yourself. I hope this book has stimulated you to further educate yourself about staying healthy and safe and looking and feeling your best. As new research and technologies evolve I will attempt to keep this information updated at my website www.saveyourface.com.

My goal in writing this book has been to teach you the truth about this important and increasingly popular topic. I have tried to present a balanced and honest presentation which includes the risks as well as the rewards of pursuing some form of facial rejuvenation as part of an over-all program of health and self improvement. Obviously, as a plastic surgeon, I believe in the value and worth of my profession and sincerely hope that what you have learned in this book will help you safely and happily achieve your goals. Good luck and good health! It is my hope that we will be able to continue this important discussion and our relationship through cyberspace. Finally, as Forrest Gump so eloquently and simply stated, "And that's all I have to say about that!"

## REFERENCES

1. Hubbs, L. Treating complications caused by non-physicians. Skin & Aging. 10: 57, 2002.
2. Phillips, K. A. The Broken Mirror: Understanding and Treating Body Dysmorphic Disorder, New York: Oxford University Press, 1986. Pp. 33.

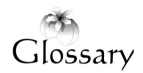

# Glossary

**ACTINIC KERATOSES-** a dry, scaling, patch of irritated skin (keratoses) caused by sun (actinic) damage to the skin. May be a precursor to skin cancer.

**AGE SPOTS-** pigmented (brown) spots on the skin seen in older people. Also called "liver spots" and "sun spots". Seen most commonly on the hands and face, areas most frequently exposed to the sun. Represent the skin's attempt to protect itself from the sun by producing pigment.

**ALTERNATIVE MEDICINE-** a wide range of healing methods not used in conventional western medicine, also described as "complimentary medicine".

**AMERICAN SOCIETY OF AESTHETIC PLASTIC SURGEONS-** A society of board certified plastic surgeons with special interest and experience in aesthetic or cosmetic plastic surgery.

**AMERICAN BOARD OF PLASTIC SURGERY-** An organization which oversees and implements the board certification process in plastic surgery.

264

**AMERICAN COUNCIL ON GRADUATE MEDICAL EDUCATION (ACGME)-** The organization which oversees and regulates the residency training programs of the various medical and surgical specialties in the United States.

**AMERICAN SOCIETY OF PLASTIC SURGERY-** A society of board certified plastic surgeons which sponsors continuing education in plastic surgery and the enforcement of ethical and professional standards. Board certification in plastic surgery is required for membership.

**ANTIOXIDANT-** Any compound or element which prevents oxidation by free radicals.

**ANTIOXIDANT VITAMINS-** Vitamins which prevent oxidation by scavenging or removing free radicals.

**ATOM-** the smallest unit into which matter can be divided and still retain the characteristic properties of the element.

**ATROPHY-** Wasting away or loss of

**AUTOIMMUNE RESPONSE-** A response of the body's immune system in which the body's immune defense system attacks the host body. Rheumatoid arthritis is an example.

**BODY DYSMORPHIC DISORDER-** A psychological illness characterized by an obsessive preoccupation with an imagined physical defect.

**BASAL CELL CARCINOMA-** A skin cancer arising in the basal layer (the deep layer) of the epithelium. More common in sun exposed areas and in people with less genetically determined sun protection i.e. fair skinned individuals.

**BLEACHING AGENTS-** Topical solutions which when applied to the skin, bleach or lighten brown pigmented areas.

**BLEPHAROPLASTY-** A plastic surgical operation performed on the eyelids to remove excess skin and fat in order to restore a youthful appearance to the eyelids. Also known as eyelids "tuck".

**BOARD CERTIFIED PHYSICIAN-** A physician who has successfully completed an approved residency training program and a certifying examination in a medical or surgical specialty approved by the American Council on Graduate Medical Education (ACGME).

**BROW PTOSIS-** Sagging of the eyebrow.

**BROW LIFT-** A plastic surgical operation to lift the brow and restore a youthful appearance to the forehead and eyes.

**BROWN SPOTS-** Brown or pigmented spots on the skin caused by sun exposure and aging. Also called age spots, liver spots, and sun spots.

**BUNNY LINES-** Wrinkles around the base of the nose between the eyes caused by the pull of the muscles of facial expression.

**CELL-** The smallest structural unit of living matter that is able to function independently.

**CELL MEMBRANE-** A thin layer that forms the outer boundary of a living cell.

**CHEMICAL PEEL-** A procedure in which an irritant such as an acid is applied to the skin to remove the outer layers of skin cells and injure the deeper layers of the skin to stimulate new collagen production.

**CORONARY ARTERY DISEASE-** The accumulation of fat laden plaques within the walls of the blood vessels in the heart which interrupt blood flow to the heart muscle and cause "heart attacks".

**CROW'S FEET-** Lines around the outside corners of the eyelids which form during facial aging. They are caused by the pull of the muscles of facial expression.

**CRUCIFEROUS VEGETABLES-** Vegetables with thick partially developed flower structures and fleshy stalks, rich in antioxidant vitamins. Broccoli and cauliflower are examples.

**CYTOKINES-** Chemical messengers released in the body after injury to a cell. They signal the elements from the blood stream to initiate the inflammatory response.

**DARK CIRCLES-** A shadow under the lower eyelid caused by aging changes beneath the skin. Frequently described as a "tired look".

**DERMIS-** The deep layer of the skin below the epidermis. Location of the collagen and elastin necessary for skin elasticity.

**DETOXIFICATION-** The process by which toxins are removed from the body. The liver plays a primary role in this process.

**DIGESTIVE ENZYME DEFICIENCY-** A condition in which inadequate digestion of food results in partially digested food acting as a foreign protein and stimulating an immune response.

**DNA-** (Deoxyribonucleic Acid) A complex organic compound found in all living cells and viruses, and is the substance which makes up genes.

**ELASTICITY-** The ability of the skin to return to its original shape after being pulled or stretched.

**ELASTIN-** A specialized form of collagen found in the dermis which is responsible for the elasticity of the skin.

**ELECTRON-** The lightest sub-atomic particle known. It carries a negative (-) electrical charge.

**EPIDERMIS-** The outer surface layer of the skin.

**EPITHELIAL CELLS-** The skin cells which make up the epidermis.

**ERBIUM LASER-** Laser with a wavelength of 2.94 microns used for facial resurfacing.

**ESTROGEN-** A class of sex hormone which primarily effects the development, maturation, and function of the female reproductive system.

**EXFOLIATION-** The process of removing the outer usually dead layers of the skin.

**EXTRINSIC AGING-** Aging changes that are precipitated or caused by factors outside of the body.

**EYELID BAGS-** Puffiness or fullness of the lower eyelids caused by the pressure of protruding fat beneath the skin of the lower eyelid.

**FACE-LIFT-** A plastic surgical operation to tighten or lift the facial skin and restore a youthful appearance to the face.

**FACIAL REJUVENATION-** The process of restoring a face to a more youthful form and appearance.

**FAT TRANSPLANTATION-** A plastic surgical procedure in which fat cells are removed from one area of the body and surgically placed into another area of the body. This procedure is most commonly performed to fill depressions or lines in the face caused by aging.

**FIBROBLAST-** A specialized cell in the body which has the ability to produce or manufacture collagen. This cell is the primary cell in the process of scar formation.

**FILLERS-** Synthetic or manufactured substances that are injected into the skin to "plump up" or fill depressions or wrinkles in the skin caused by aging.

**FREE RADICAL-** A molecule containing at least one unpaired electron (-). Free radicals can produce significant damage to the cells of the body. They are produced during the metabolism of food in the mitochondria.

**FREE RADICAL SCAVENGERS-** Substances which attach to and render harmless free radicals. Vitamin C and other antioxidant vitamins are examples.

**FROWN LINES-** Lines between the eyebrows which are accentuated during frowning and become permanent with aging. They are caused by the pull of the muscles of facial expression.

**GENE-** A structure composed of DNA which resides on the chromosome in the nucleus of the cell and determines heredity. Genes exert their influence by controlling the molecular machinery of the cell.

**GLYCATION-** The attachment of a glucose or sugar molecule to a protein, creating damage and rendering the protein ineffective.

**HEART ATTACK-** Damage to the muscle of the heart caused by interruption of blood flow to the heart. The classic symptom is chest pain. The heart attack can be fatal.

**HERNIATE-** To rupture or push through.

**HISTAMINE-** A chemical released by the mast cell during an inflammatory response. The response of the body to histamine release is dilation of the blood vessels which causes redness of the skin, watering of the eyes, and runny nose, often called an allergic response.

**HORMONE REPLACEMENT THERAPY (HRT)-** Therapy to replace the hormone estrogen after menopause.

**HUMAN GENOME PROJECT-** A research project designed to map and identify the genes located on the human chromosome. The identification of the structure of the human genes will enable scientists to synthesize genes and insert them into abnormal cells and correct genetic abnormalities which cause diseases such as diabetes.

**HUMAN GROWTH HORMONE-** A hormone responsible for growth and development in the human. Levels decrease with age and correction of deficiencies of this hormone have been associated with remarkable anti-aging effects.

**HYALURONIC ACID-** A biologically active compound called a mucopolysaccharide found in all tissues but in highest concentrations in the embryo. Present in the skin and responsible for moisture content. Decreases dramatically with aging.

**INFLAMMATION-** A response of the cells of the body to injury which releases histamine and ultimately leads to proliferation of fibroblasts and scarring.

**INFOMERCIALS-** Advertisements which purport to be providing impartial educational information but in reality are commercials designed to stimulate the recipient to buy a product.

**INFRARED LIGHT-** Light with a wavelength of 0.7-10.6 microns emitted by heat, used for night vision equipment and as an energy source for collagen remodeling.

**INSULIN-** A hormone released by the pancreas essential for the breakdown of starches, the entrance of carbohydrates into the bloodstream, and the metabolism of sugars and fats.

**INTESTINAL DYSBIOSIS-** The imbalance of the normal bacterial flora present in the large intestine caused by the consumption of antibiotics both prescription and in the food supply.

**INTRINSIC AGING-** Aging of the body caused by internal or inherent factors in the body.

**IPL-** (Intense Pulsed Light) Light generated by a flash lamp in a machine through a lens designed to allow through specific therapeutic wavelengths of light used to remove pigment, blood vessels, and to stimulate new collagen production in the skin.

**LASER-** A machine designed to produce an intense beam of light which is monochromatic (one color) and coherent (stays together). Laser stands for "light amplification by stimulated emission of radiation". Energy, usually electrical is supplied to a tube containing a gas. The electrical energy forces electrons away from the atoms of the gas in the tube, the electrons are accelerated by bouncing off of mirrors in the tube, and are released from the tube as powerful light beams.

**LASER RESURFACING-** A plastic surgical procedure during which a laser beam is used to ablate or remove old damaged skin from the face and injure the dermis so that new skin, new epithelium and new dermis with new dermal collagen is formed, and wrinkles and sun damage are removed.

**LED-** (Light Emitting Diode) The red blinking light you see on your remote control and microwave.

**LIPSTICK LINES-** Vertical lines in the skin around the lips caused by the pull of the muscles of facial expression, and more noticeable with aging. Terribly accentuated by smoking cigarettes.

**LOSS OF ELASTICITY-** A failure of the skin to return to its normal shape after being pulled or stretched.

**MACROPHAGE-** A cell which responds to inflammation by migrating into the injured area and ingesting and removing damaged cells. Once damaged cells are removed the macrophage transforms into a fibroblast and produces collagen and a scar.

**MALAR FAT PAD-** A pad of fat high in the cheek on top of the cheek bone in youth responsible for the "chubby cheeks" of children. With facial aging and loss of elasticity the fat pad falls creating a hollow where it used to be. The hollow contributes to the tear trough deformity.

**MARIONETTE LINES-** Deep lines below the corner of the mouth caused by sagging of the cheek skin with aging of the face.

**MAST CELL-** A cell involved in the initiation of the inflammatory response. Following injury mast cells migrate into the injured area and release chemicals such as histamine that begin the inflammatory response.

**MELANOMA-** A malignant form of skin cancer arising from the pigment cells of the skin. Intense sun exposure especially to fair skinned children increases the risk of this cancer in later life.

**MELATONIN-** A hormone secreted by the pineal gland in the brain that controls sleep-wake cycles. This hormone is believed by some to have anti-aging properties.

**MENOPAUSE-** Final cessation of menstruation, ending female fertility.

**MICROLASERPEEL®-** A superficial type of laser skin peel performed with the Erbium laser. The depth of the skin peel is usually 20-40 microns.

**MICRODERMABRASION-** A "no down time" skin peel performed by superficially abrading the skin with a device which passes silica particles across skin which is held tight to the device by vacuum pressure. The depth of the peel is usually 8 microns.

**MICROPEEL®-** A superficial skin peel performed by mechanically scraping dead skin off of the face using a scalpel, a technique called dermaplaning. After dermaplaning a dilute solution of AHAs are applied to the skin. Depth of the procedure is approximately 5 microns.

**MICRON-** A unit of measurement that is one thousandth of a millimeter or one millionth of a meter.

**MITOCHONDRION-** A small structure in the cytoplasm of the cell that is responsible for the production of energy in the cell from the metabolism of food. Free radicals are generated during this process.

**MOLECULE-** The smallest particle of a substance that retains all the properties of the substance and is composed of one or more atoms.

**MUSCLES OF FACIAL EXPRESSION-** The muscles of the face responsible for facial expressions during acts such as smiling, frowning, crying, etc. With facial aging the pull of these muscles creates wrinkles or lines on the face called the lines of facial expression.

**NASAL-LABIAL FOLD-** A fold of cheek skin hanging over a line that runs from the outside corner of the nostril to the corner of the mouth.

**NASAL- LABIAL FOLD LINE-** The line beneath the nasal-labial fold caused by the pull of the smile muscles.

**"NO DOWN TIME" PROCEDURE-** Term used in this book to refer to facial rejuvenation procedures that produce minimal or no redness or discomfort and do not require a recovery period. Thus a person may have this type of procedure and return to work or other normal daily activity immediately.

**NON-ABLATIVE THERAPY-** Used in this book to describe a facial rejuvenation therapy which does not ablate or remove the superficial layer of the skin, the epidermis, and thus does not create an open wound which would require post operative care.

**PIGMENT CELLS-** Cells of the skin which produce pigment or color, also called melanocytes. These cells are responsible for skin color, tanning, and brown spots, age spots, and sunspots.

**PLASTIC SURGEON-** A surgeon certified by the American Board of Plastic Surgery to perform plastic surgical operations.

**PLASTIC SURGERY-** An ACGME recognized, board certifiable, field of specialization in surgery. Board certified plastic surgeons perform surgical operations to correct congenital and acquired deformities of the face, hands, breast, and body. The word plastic comes from the Greek word plastics which means to mold or give form.

**PLASTIC SURGERY ADDICTION-** A lay term used to describe body dysmorphic disorder, a the condition manifested by a person having multiple plastic surgeries to correct an imagined or minor physical deformity.

**PLATYSMAL BAND-** A band or fold of skin hanging below the chin, running from the chin down into the neck.

**PROCESSED FOODS-** Foods that have been altered from their natural form by chemical or mechanical manipulation or the addition of preservatives or other compounds.

**Proton-** A particle that is identical with the nucleus of the hydrogen atom, that along with neutrons is a constituent of all other atomic nuclei, that carries a positive charge numerically equal to the charge of an electron.

**Radiofrequency-** Radiant energy of a certain frequency, above 10 microns up to thousands of meters. Used to transmit radio and television but also used in specialized machines to tighten skin.

**Raise a red flag-** A warning usually of impending danger, for example, red flags are raised in costal areas to warn of an approaching hurricane.

**Refined starches-** Carbohydrates such as sugar and flour that have been chemically or mechanically altered or processed to change them from their natural state.

**Resident-** A house officer or "resident physician" affiliated with a hospital for the purpose of clinical training. Formerly residents actually lived at the hospital. However, today residents live at home, and sleep in the hospitals only when on night call and the responsibilities of patient care require it.

**RetinA®-** A retinoid used as a topical skin solution to stimulate new cell formation by the epidermis and the production of new collagen in the dermis

**RETINOIDS-** A class of topical skin drugs, derived from Vitamin A used for treating acne, psoriasis, sun damage and facial aging. These drugs are keratolytic, meaning they remove keratin, the compound contained in superficial skin cells.

**RETINOLS-** A retinoid that is a precursor to tretinoin (Retin A). Retinols are not as powerful as tretinoin and can be used in patients with sensitive skin.

**RHYTIDECTOMY-** The medical term for a face-lift. Rhytid means loose skin, – ectomy means to cut out or remove.

**ROSACEA-** A skin disorder manifested by a pink or red flush and dilated blood vessels in the skin of the face around the nose and on the cheeks.

**SCAR-** Fibrous tissue replacing normal tissue as a result of injury or disease.

**SKIN CANER-** A cancer arising in the skin.

**SKIN LAXITY-** Looseness of the skin caused by loss of elasticity.

**SKIN PEEL-** A procedure during which the outer layers of the skin are removed or peeled away, usually by the application of an acid or a laser.

**SKIN TYPE-** The genetically determined characteristics of skin, including color, thickness, and susceptibility to sun burn, and associated with characteristic hair and eye color.

**SKINCEUTICALS-** A term used to refer to topical solutions applied to the skin for the purpose of exerting a pharmacological effect, also called Cosmaceutical.

**SMILE LINES-** Lines around the mouth and on the cheeks created during the act of smiling.

**SOLAR ELASTOSIS-** A pathological diagnosis made upon microscopic examination of the skin manifested by the accumulation of damaged elastin fibers in the deeper layers of the dermis. This condition is caused by damage to the dermal collagen and elastin by the UV (ultraviolet) rays of the sun and by aging.

**SQUAMOUS CELL CARCINOMA-** A skin cancer consisting of the epithelial cells of the skin.

**STATIN DRUGS-** Drugs used to lower blood cholesterol.

**STROKE-** A medical illness caused by loss of blood supply to the brain that can result in paralysis, other neurological symptoms or death.

**SUN DAMAGED SKIN-** Skin that has been damaged by long term exposure to the sun that results in wrinkles, brown spots, actinic keratoses, and dry skin.

**SUPRATARSAL FOLD-** A curved line on the upper eyelid that appears between 8 and 12 millimeters above the eyelashes.

**TARGET SPECIFIC PHOTOTHERMOLYSIS-** The destruction of a specific target by heat produced by light energy, most commonly a laser.

**TEAR TROUGH DEFORMITY-** A line or trough running from the corner of the eye near the nose down and out to the side of the face across the cheek.

**TELANGIECTASIA-** A collection of small dilated blood vessels which appear as a red spot on the skin, most commonly around the nose and on the cheek and chin.

**TELOMERASE-** An enzyme that mediates the repair of the telomere.

**TELOMERE-** The end portion of a chromosome that controls the number of times a cell can divide.

**TESTOSTERONE-** The most potent naturally occurring male or androgenic sex hormone produced primarily by the testes, which affects the development, maturation and function of the male reproductive system.

**THYROID HORMONE-** A hormone produced by the thyroid gland that has profound effects on the metabolic rate of the body.

**TIME URGENCY-** Having too much to do in too little time.

**TOPICAL AGENTS-** Medications applied directly to the skin as opposed to those taken internally by mouth.

**TRANSCONJUNCTIVAL BLEPHAROPLASTY-** An eyelid rejuvenation operation performed through a small incision inside the eyelid so that there is no visible scar left on the outside of the eyelid skin.

**ULTRAVIOLET LIGHT-** Light with a wavelength less than 0.4 microns that occupies from violet on the visible light spectrum down to the x-ray portion of the electromagnetic spectrum. Ultraviolet radiation comes from sunlight and is divided into 3 bands, UVA, UVB, and UVC (which does not reach the earth). UVB has the most profound effect on the skin causing sunburn, aging changes, and skin cancer. UVA has similar but less intense damaging effects on the skin.

**VITAMIN-** One of a group of organic substances present in minute amounts in natural foodstuffs that are essential to normal metabolism. Significant deficiencies of some vitamins can cause serious medical illness.

**WORRY LINES-** Transverse lines which run across the forehead accentuated by the facial expression associated with worry or stress. Caused by the pull of muscles of facial expression.

**WRINKLE-** As used in this book, a linear depression or crease in the skin associated with aging particularly when present in the facial skin. Factors which contribute to the formation of wrinkles in the skin are damage to and atrophy of the collagen and elastin in the dermis, loss of skin elasticity, atrophy or loss of subcutaneous fat, and the pull of the muscles of facial expression.

# Index

_your_

# SAVE ^ FACE

## ORDER FORM

Send Payment to:

**PEACH PUBLICATIONS**

25 Fairhaven Road

Concord, MA 01742

Please allow 4-6 weeks for delivery

Outside the US 6-8 weeks for delivery

Bill My: ☐ VISA

☐ MASTERCARD

Card#_____

Expiration Date_____

Signature _____

---

**BILL TO:** ☐ SAME AS SHIPPING ADDRESS

Name:_____

Address:_____

City:_____ State:_____ Zip Code:_____

Day Time Phone:_____ Email:_____

---

**SHIP TO:**

Name:_____

Address:_____

City:_____ State:_____ Zip Code:_____

Day Time Phone:_____ Email:_____

---

**NUMBER OF BOOKS AT $19.95 EACH** . . . . . . . . . . . . [        ]

**APPLICABLE SALES TAX**

**Postage & Handling ($3.00 per book within the US)** . . . . [        ]

**($5.00 per book outside the US)** . . . [        ]

**TOTAL AMOUNT DUE** . . . . . . . . . . . . . . . . . . . . [        ]

_Prices Subject to Change Without Notice_

# THE END?

# NO!

## JUST THE BEGINNING...

ANTI-AGING DISCOVERIES ARE ON-GOING.
CONTINUE TO "SAVE YOUR FACE"
BY VISITING OUR WEB PAGE AT

## www.saveyourface.com

- **ASK DR. SECKEL**
- **LASTEST ANTI-AGING UPDATES**
- **ON-LINE NEWSLETTERS**

To show our appreciation, subscribe to our
"Save Your Face" Newsletter and
receive the first issue

# FREE